Updates in Surgery

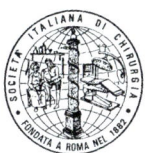

The aim of this series is to provide informative updates on hot topics in the areas of breast, endocrine, and abdominal surgery, surgical oncology, and coloproctology, and on new surgical techniques such as robotic surgery, laparoscopy, and minimally invasive surgery. Readers will find detailed guidance on patient selection, performance of surgical procedures, and avoidance of complications. In addition, a range of other important aspects are covered, from the role of new imaging tools to the use of combined treatments and postoperative care.

The topics addressed by volumes in the series Updates in Surgery have been selected for their broad significance in collaboration with the Italian Society of Surgery. Each volume will assist surgical residents and fellows and practicing surgeons in reaching appropriate treatment decisions and achieving optimal outcomes. The series will also be highly relevant for surgical researchers.

Vincenzo Landolfi • Salvatore Tolone
Editors

Functional Diseases of the Esophagus

Pathophysiology, Diagnosis and Surgical Technique

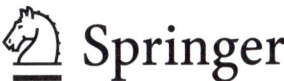

Editors
Vincenzo Landolfi
UOC General Surgery
AORN San Giuseppe Moscati
Avellino, Italy

Salvatore Tolone
UOC General, Mininvasive, Oncological
and Bariatric Surgery
University of Campania "Luigi Vanvitelli"
Naples, Italy

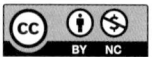

ISSN 2280-9848   ISSN 2281-0854   (electronic)
Updates in Surgery
ISBN 978-3-031-90569-8   ISBN 978-3-031-90570-4   (eBook)
https://doi.org/10.1007/978-3-031-90570-4

The publication and the distribution of this volume have been supported by the Italian Society of Surgery.

The Editors of the volume and the Italian Society of Surgery would like to thank Becton, Dickinson Italia S.p.A. for their unconditional contribution, which made it possible to publish this book under the Open Access model.

© The Editor(s) (if applicable) and The Author(s) 2026. This book is an open access publication.

Open Access This book is licensed under the terms of the Creative Commons Attribution-NonCommercial 4.0 International License (http://creativecommons.org/licenses/by-nc/4.0/), which permits any noncommercial use, sharing, adaptation, distribution and reproduction in any medium or format, as long as you give appropriate credit to the original author(s) and the source, provide a link to the Creative Commons license and indicate if changes were made.
The images or other third party material in this book are included in the book's Creative Commons license, unless indicated otherwise in a credit line to the material. If material is not included in the book's Creative Commons license and your intended use is not permitted by statutory regulation or exceeds the permitted use, you will need to obtain permission directly from the copyright holder.
This work is subject to copyright. All commercial rights are reserved by the author(s), whether the whole or part of the material is concerned, specifically the rights of translation, reprinting, reuse of illustrations, recitation, broadcasting, reproduction on microfilms or in any other physical way, and transmission or information storage and retrieval, electronic adaptation, computer software, or by similar or dissimilar methodology now known or hereafter developed. Regarding these commercial rights a non-exclusive license has been granted to the publisher.
The use of general descriptive names, registered names, trademarks, service marks, etc. in this publication does not imply, even in the absence of a specific statement, that such names are exempt from the relevant protective laws and regulations and therefore free for general use.
The publisher, the authors and the editors are safe to assume that the advice and information in this book are believed to be true and accurate at the date of publication. Neither the publisher nor the authors or the editors give a warranty, expressed or implied, with respect to the material contained herein or for any errors or omissions that may have been made. The publisher remains neutral with regard to jurisdictional claims in published maps and institutional affiliations.

This Springer imprint is published by the registered company Springer Nature Switzerland AG
The registered company address is: Gewerbestrasse 11, 6330 Cham, Switzerland

If disposing of this product, please recycle the paper.

Foreword

It is an honor to introduce this very important book on esophageal functional diseases. For some time, both I and the Executive Board of the Italian Society of Surgery had felt the need to fine-tune this theme, partly because during the over 30 years of the Society's Monographs this topic had never been addressed, and partly because this pathological condition has seen a number of conceptual progressions, technical evolutions, and outcome improvements. For these reasons I want to thank and congratulate the editors, Profs. Vincenzo Landolfi and Salvatore Tolone, and the authors on the extensive work they have done on this topic.

The volume covers in 21 chapters all the aspects of functional esophageal diseases, from the history and treatment of these disorders to the new insights into the anatomy, physiology, epidemiology, and pathophysiology. The diagnostic aspects of radiological, endoscopic, and manometric investigations, pH-metry and monitoring, and neuromuscular tests are all beautifully described.

All the nosological frameworks are comprehensively discussed: GERD, esophagitis and Barret's esophagus, achalasia, pharyngoesophageal and epiphrenic diverticula, and diffuse esophageal spasm are magisterially described by real experts. An important in-depth focus is dedicated to GERD. For this very frequent disease, not only the surgical antireflux procedures, treatment of antireflux surgery complications, and endoscopic treatment are addressed but medical management, diet, and rehabilitation are covered in detail in dedicated sections.

I would like to express my gratitude to the editors and authors for realizing this monograph, which with its high scientific level maintains the high standard of the Biennial Reports of the Italian Society of Surgery, and will be a reference for the surgical community worldwide.

Rome, Italy Massimo Carlini
September 2025

Preface

Over the last two decades, the conceptual understanding of functional disorders of the esophagus has undergone a profound transformation. Advances in diagnostic technology, refinement of pathophysiological models, and the evolution of therapeutic strategies—both medical and surgical—have redefined how we classify, interpret, and manage these disorders. It is within this dynamic and challenging context that this book was conceived and strongly desired.
The esophagus is far more than a simple conduit between the mouth and the stomach; it is a highly coordinated, neuromuscular organ whose dysfunction can result in a wide range of debilitating symptoms—chest pain, dysphagia, regurgitation, and heartburn among them—that significantly impair patients' quality of life. Esophageal pathology, including gastroesophageal reflux disease (GERD), achalasia, esophagogastric junction outflow obstruction (EGJ-OO), diffuse esophageal spasm, hypercontractile esophagus, remain diagnostically and therapeutically changeling. They are frequently under-recognized or misdiagnosed for a long time, especially when endoscopy or imaging show some structural anomaly. In these cases, pathophysiology must be inferred from motility studies with high-resolution manometry (HRM), pH-monitoring (wireless or catheter-based with or without impedance), and emerging techniques—an interpretive art that is still evolving.

This book offers the most comprehensive and current synthesis of knowledge on the topic of functional esophageal diseases. It reflects the work and collaboration of a team of experts in gastroenterology, gastrointestinal physiology, and foregut surgery. Our contributors have been carefully selected not only for their expertise and scientific contributions to the field but also for their ability to translate complex concepts into clinically applicable insights. Their collective experience, drawn from academic and high-volume centers across the globe, ensures that the content presented in this volume is both evidence-based and reflective of contemporary best practice.

The book is divided into multiple sections, each focusing on a distinct yet interrelated aspect of esophageal functional pathology. We begin with a foundational exploration of esophageal physiology and motility, outlining the neuroanatomical and biomechanical principles that underlie normal esophageal function. These chapters lay the groundwork for a nuanced understanding of functional disorders, as disturbances in these mechanisms give rise to the various clinical syndromes discussed later.

Subsequent chapters delve into the modern classification of esophageal motility disorders, particularly as defined by the Chicago Classification—now in its 4.0

iteration—and discuss its strengths, limitations, and clinical implications. Special attention is given to the role of HRM, which has revolutionized our approach to diagnosis, enabling clinicians to visualize and interpret esophageal pressure topography with unprecedented clarity.

We include detailed parts on other diagnostic modalities such as pH-impedance monitoring, functional luminal imaging probe (FLIP), and barium esophagography. These tools provide complementary information and, when used in concert, can dramatically enhance diagnostic accuracy and therapeutic planning.

Treatment modalities are covered in depth, reflecting the interdisciplinary nature of care required for these patients. Pharmacological therapies, including the role of calcium channel blockers, nitrates, neuromodulators, and emerging targeted therapies, are presented with critical analysis of their efficacy and side-effect profiles. Non-pharmacological interventions, such as dietary strategies, are also discussed, recognizing the biopsychosocial model increasingly embraced in functional gastrointestinal disorders.

Surgical and endoscopic innovations have significantly reshaped the therapeutic landscape. Chapters dedicated to minimally invasive approaches as well as endoscopic techniques provide both technical detail and outcome data. These discussions emphasize the importance of careful patient selection, preoperative evaluation, and long-term follow-up, particularly in complex or recurrent cases.

The publication of this book arrives at a critical juncture in the care of patients with esophageal functional disorders. As our understanding deepens, so too does the appreciation for the complexity and individuality of these conditions. The need for personalized medicine—guided by physiology, symptomatology, patient preference, and long-term outcomes—has never been greater. We hope this book will not only serve as a reference for current best practices but also as a catalyst for further inquiry, innovation, and collaboration.

We envision this work as a valuable resource for a wide audience: gastroenterologists, surgeons, residents, fellows, nurse specialists, and researchers alike. Whether used as a textbook for training, a reference for clinical decision-making, or a platform for academic discussion, we trust it will enrich your understanding and support your work in delivering high-quality, compassionate care to patients affected by these challenging disorders.

We deeply want to thank the *Società Italiana di Chirurgia* (SIC, Italian Society of Surgery), the President, and all the Committee Members for giving us the possibility to start this project and to present it in its final form during the 2025 Annual Meeting as a Biennial Lecture.

Finally, we extend our deepest gratitude to all the authors, reviewers, and production staff whose dedication and expertise have made this book possible. Their commitment to advancing the field of esophageal functional disorders—and to improving the lives of patients—resonates on every page.

Avellino, Italy	Vincenzo Landolfi
Naples, Italy	Salvatore Tolone
September 2025	

Contents

1. **History of Esophageal Functional Diseases and Their Treatment** 1
   Natale Di Martino, Luigi Marano, Luigi Monaco,
   and Francesco Torelli

2. **Esophageal Anatomy and Physiology. Epidemiology
   and Pathophysiology of Functional Disorders** 13
   Giovanni Aldinio, Beatrice Marinoni, Marina Coletta,
   and Roberto Penagini

3. **Radiological Evaluation of Functional Diseases
   of the Esophagus** 23
   Alfonso Reginelli, Vittorio Patanè, and Roberto Grassi

4. **Functional Motor Disorders of the Esophagus** 33
   Nicola de Bortoli and Irene Solinas

5. **Esophageal pH and pH-Impedance Monitoring** 45
   Edoardo Vincenzo Savarino and Luisa Bertin

6. **New Techniques of Endoscopy**................................. 55
   Pier Alberto Testoni and Sabrina Testoni

7. **Hypotonic Lower Esophageal Sphincter and Hiatal Hernia:
   Clinical Symptoms and Diagnosis** 69
   Stefano Siboni and Marco Sozzi

8. **Neuromuscular Diagnosis by Esophageal Tests** 77
   Pierfrancesco Visaggi

9. **Esophagitis and Barrett's Esophagus** 83
   Giuseppe Galloro, Rosa Maione, and Alessia Chini

10. **Medical Management** 93
    Marzio Frazzoni and Leonardo Frazzoni

11. **Diet** 101
    Antonella Santonicola, Ida de Micco, Luigi Schiavo,
    and Paola Iovino

12	**Rehabilitation** 109	
	Adriana Maria Landolfi	
13	**Surgical Antireflux Procedures** 115	
	Vincenzo Landolfi and Salvatore Tolone	
14	**Endoscopic Treatment of Gastroesophageal Reflux Disease**......... 123	
	Guido Costamagna and Cristina Ciuffini	
15	**Treatment of Antireflux Surgery Complications** 131	
	Mario Morino and Elettra Ugliono	
16	**Obesity, Bariatric Surgery and Gastroesophageal Reflux Disease** 141	
	Salvatore Tolone and Ludovico Docimo	
17	**Clinical Evaluation, Etiology and Classification of Esophageal Achalasia** 147	
	Mario Costantini and Andrea Costantini	
18	**Heller Myotomy and Antireflux Techniques**...................... 157	
	Renato Salvador, Andrea Costantini, Matteo Santangelo, and Salvatore Tolone	
19	**Pharyngoesophageal Diverticula**............................... 171	
	Luigi Bonavina	
20	**Epiphrenic Diverticula** 177	
	Lavinia Alessandra Barbieri, Silvia Battaglia, Agnese Carresi, Francesco Puccetti, Ugo Elmore, and Riccardo Rosati	
21	**Diffuse Esophageal Spasm** 185	
	Alberto Aiolfi and Davide Bona	

History of Esophageal Functional Diseases and Their Treatment

Natale Di Martino, Luigi Marano, Luigi Monaco, and Francesco Torelli

1.1 Introduction

Esophageal functional diseases, such as achalasia, gastroesophageal reflux disease (GERD), and diffuse esophageal spasm, significantly impact health by causing symptoms like dysphagia, chest pain, and heartburn. Unlike structural abnormalities, these conditions stem from esophageal motility dysfunction, posing unique challenges in diagnosis and treatment [1]. The historical evolution of treating these disorders, shaped by anatomical difficulties, technological advances, and clinical knowledge, offers insights into current practices.

The esophagus's location, minimal blood supply, and lack of a protective serous layer made early surgical intervention difficult. Perforation often led to fatal infections, delaying surgical success [2]. The first recorded esophageal surgery dates to ancient Egypt, documented in the Edwin Smith Papyrus (1600 BCE), though significant progress remained slow for centuries [3].

In the 12th century, Avenzoar suggested using cannulas for patients unable to swallow, an early recognition of esophageal dysfunction. By the Renaissance, advancements in anatomical dissection led to some progress. Richard Wiseman

---

N. Di Martino · F. Torelli
Department of Surgery, University of Campania "Luigi Vanvitelli", Naples, Italy
e-mail: natale.dimartino@unicampania.it; francesco.torelli@unicampania.it

L. Marano (✉)
Department of Medicine, Academy of Applied Medical and Social Sciences-AMiSNS: Akademia Medycznych I Spolecznych Nauk Stosowanych, Elbląg, Poland

Department of General Surgery and Surgical Oncology, "Saint Wojciech" Hospital, "Nicolaus Copernicus" Health Center, Gdańsk, Poland
e-mail: l.marano@amisns.edu.pl

L. Monaco
Department of General Surgery, Villa Esther Clinic, Pineta Grande Hospital, Avellino, Italy
e-mail: info@luigimonaco.it

recommended suturing esophageal tears in 1676, while others, like Johann Dietrich Purmann, advocated for natural healing [4].

By the 19th century, surgery began advancing more rapidly. In 1805, Vigardonne deemed esophagotomy safe, and by 1867 David Cheever documented growing success in the procedure. By 1880, Samuel Gross reported numerous successful surgeries, challenging earlier fears about esophageal operations [5].

The 20th century saw a major leap in esophageal surgery with innovations like aseptic techniques, intratracheal anesthesia, and antibiotics. Pioneers like Jan Mikulicz-Radecki and Ferdinand Sauerbruch advanced respiratory control, crucial for thoracic and esophageal procedures. Radiologic imaging, esophageal manometry, and pH monitoring improved diagnostic precision, while advances in anesthesia and respiratory management made surgery safer and more effective [6]. By the mid-20th century, surgeons like Chevalier Jackson and anesthesiologists like Ralph Waters and Sir Ivan Magill enhanced laryngoscopy and intubation techniques [7]. World War II experiences further advanced emergency care, improving surgical outcomes [8].

In recent decades, esophageal surgery has been transformed by minimally invasive techniques (MIS), including endoscopic, laparoscopic, and robotic approaches [9]. Robotic systems, in particular, have made complex esophageal surgeries more feasible. MIS has shown numerous benefits, such as reduced complications, faster recovery, and shorter hospital stays, making it a preferred choice, especially for younger patients [10]. These advancements continue to provide better treatment options, shaping the future of esophageal surgery.

1.2 Esophageal Achalasia Surgery: Historical Perspectives

Esophageal achalasia is one of the oldest documented esophageal disorders, first described in detail by Thomas Willis in 1674. He observed a patient suffering from chronic vomiting due to an obstruction at the esophageal entrance (the cardia) and devised a primitive tool using whale bone and a sponge to push food into the stomach, allowing the patient to survive for 15 years. This was the earliest documented treatment of esophageal achalasia [11].

In 1821, Purton added further documentation, and by 1878, Zenker and Von Ziemssen expanded clinical understanding with 17 cases of "cardiospasm." In 1887, J.C. Russell introduced a silk-covered inflatable balloon attached to a bougie to dilate the esophagus, marking an early non-surgical treatment. However, true surgical breakthroughs came in the early 20th century [12].

1.2.1 Early Surgical Developments

Surgical attempts to treat achalasia began in 1903 with esophagogastrostomy procedures aimed at improving esophageal emptying. Surgeons like Marwedel and Wendel developed various techniques, including side-to-side esophagogastrostomies and

U-shaped incisions along the esophagus and stomach. Unfortunately, these often caused severe reflux, leading to esophagitis and stenosis, and fell out of favor by the 1940s [3].

On April 14, 1913, Ernst Heller performed the first effective extramucosal cardiomyotomy, which involved cutting both the anterior and posterior esophageal muscles to relieve the obstruction at the lower esophageal sphincter [13]. This procedure marked a major milestone in esophageal surgery, laying the foundation for modern achalasia treatment. Earlier efforts by surgeons like Mikulicz and Reisinger focused on dilation, but Heller's myotomy became the first truly effective solution [14].

Although Heller's procedure resolved muscle non-relaxation, it introduced the risk of postoperative reflux. To address this, surgeons began incorporating anti-reflux techniques. In 1962, Dor proposed an anterior hemifundoplication to prevent reflux and protect the mucosa during surgery [15]. Later, Toupet introduced a posterior hemifundoplication, balancing the resolution of dysphagia with the need to prevent reflux, a persistent challenge in achalasia surgery [16].

1.2.2 Modern Surgical Techniques and the Minimally Invasive Era

The late 20th century saw significant advancements in surgical techniques, particularly with the advent of minimally invasive procedures. Laparoscopic surgery emerged as a transformative approach, reducing patient recovery times and minimizing postoperative discomfort. In 1991, A. Cuschieri performed the first laparoscopic cardiomyotomy [17], followed by C. Pellegrini in 1992, who adapted the laparoscopic approach to replicate traditional open surgical outcomes [18]. These developments revolutionized the treatment of foregut disorders, including achalasia.

In recent years, robotic surgery has further refined these techniques. First described in a 2001 case report by Melvin et al. [19], it was demonstrated that robotic-assisted cardiomyotomy may reduce the risk of esophageal perforation compared to laparoscopic methods. Although the long-term superiority of robotic approaches is still debated, these technological innovations continue to advance surgical precision and safety [20].

1.2.3 Pathophysiological Understanding and Technological Advances: The Contribution of the Neapolitan Surgical School

The understanding of achalasia's pathophysiology advanced significantly during the 20th century. Early pathological studies by Rake in 1925 and Hurst in 1927 identified the degeneration of ganglion cells in Auerbach's plexus as a key contributing factor to the condition, although the precise etiology remained elusive [21]. Hurst's description of the distal esophagus's failure to relax offered a clearer understanding of the disorder, and his introduction of mercury-filled bougies for dilation became a standardized non-surgical treatment [22]. Later, Maloney refined these bougies by adding sharper tips for improved efficacy [10].

Manometric studies, which began with Kronecker and Meltzer in 1883, were instrumental in revealing the physiological underpinnings of achalasia [23]. After World War II, further investigations by Kramer, Ingelfinger, and others confirmed that Heller's myotomy effectively reduced esophageal pressure, solidifying its place in achalasia treatment [24].

Achalasia is now recognized as a disorder of the esophagus's motor function, likely influenced by immune-mediated dysfunction. It is characterized by impaired relaxation of the esophagogastric junction (EGJ) and a lack of peristalsis during swallowing. These pathological changes lead to functional obstruction at the EGJ, resulting in dysphagia and regurgitation [25]. Therapeutic interventions, including pneumatic dilation, laparoscopic Heller myotomy, and peroral endoscopic myotomy (POEM), aim to reduce the lower esophageal sphincter pressure and improve esophageal clearance, thus alleviating symptoms and improving patient quality of life [26].

Among these, surgical intervention has proven the most effective. Our team, in collaboration with the University of Amsterdam, conducted experimental studies to explore this further. Using intraoperative computerized manometry, we demonstrated that a myotomy restricted to the esophageal portion of the lower esophageal sphincter (LES) did not significantly affect pressure. However, when the gastric fibers were dissected for 2–3 cm along the anterior gastric wall, LES pressure dropped substantially, emphasizing the importance of including the gastric fibers in the procedure to avoid recurrent dysphagia [27].

While laparoscopic surgery has become the preferred approach due to its favorable outcomes, it has limitations, such as two-dimensional vision and restricted movement, which can affect surgical precision. Robotic-assisted surgery offers enhanced three-dimensional visualization and greater dexterity, potentially reducing complications like esophageal perforation [28]. Though promising, these techniques still face challenges, including a recurrence rate of symptoms in about 10–25% of patients. The European Achalasia Trial, which compared laparoscopic Heller myotomy and pneumatic dilation, showed high success rates, though these declined slightly over time, underscoring the complexity of long-term management [29].

One ongoing debate concerns the optimal length of the myotomy. Some advocate for limiting the myotomy to the lower esophagus to preserve part of the LES and reduce the risk of postoperative reflux. However, most experts recommend extending the myotomy 4–6 cm on the esophagus and 1–2 cm onto the stomach, accompanied by an anti-reflux procedure [30]. Precision surgery, tailored to each patient's anatomical features, is gaining traction as a future approach to better manage achalasia.

Managing a functional disorder like achalasia through mechanical means requires a deep understanding of esophageal anatomy and its pathophysiology. Our group was among the first in Italy to use intraoperative esophageal manometry

(IOM) routinely in 1972, a technique developed concurrently by Hill in the United States [31]. IOM allows surgeons to adjust intraoperatively based on real-time pressure measurements, ensuring full ablation of the LES high-pressure zone (HPZ). Several studies, including our own, have demonstrated that a complete myotomy extending into the gastric sling fibers significantly reduces LES pressure, which is essential for long-term success.

Despite its widespread adoption, the value of IOM remains debated due to conflicting results in the literature. Some researchers question its predictive value, while others argue that it is critical for guiding surgical decisions [32]. During Heller myotomy, IOM offers objective feedback on LES pressure reduction, helping ensure that no residual muscle fibers remain in the HPZ, which could cause symptom recurrence. Our studies found that, even with visual inspection and intraoperative endoscopy, incomplete myotomies occurred in about 15% of cases, particularly in the distal portion [31]. This underscores the importance of using IOM as an additional tool for ensuring surgical success.

Recent anatomical studies have shed light on the structural components of the LES, particularly the role of the gastric sling and semicircular clasp fibers in maintaining the HPZ. These findings suggest that a limited myotomy targeting the clasp fibers may relieve obstruction while preserving the reflux barrier, whereas a more extensive myotomy may require an anti-reflux procedure to prevent postoperative complications [33].

In our study of 150 achalasia patients, computerized manometry confirmed the effectiveness of a calibrated laparoscopic Heller myotomy. Preoperative LES pressure averaged 37.7 mmHg and, after complete myotomy, it dropped by over 90%. These findings support the need for a comprehensive myotomy extending approximately 5–6 cm on the esophagus and 3–3.5 cm onto the stomach for optimal outcomes [34].

In conclusion, our research underscores the importance of a calibrated, personalized surgical approach to achalasia management. Precision surgery, guided by intraoperative manometry, represents a key advancement in improving outcomes for patients, reducing the risk of symptom recurrence, and providing a foundation for the future of personalized care in achalasia treatment.

1.3 A Historical Overview of Esophageal Diverticula and Associated Surgical Interventions

Esophageal diverticula, along with achalasia, are classified as motility disorders of the esophagus. The earliest documentation of a pharyngo-esophageal pulsion diverticulum dates back to 1767, when Abraham Ludlow from Bristol, UK, described it in his publication titled *A Case of Obstructed Deglutition from a Preternatural Dilatation Formed in the Pharynx* [35].

In 1877, Friedrich Albert von Zenker and von Ziemssen were the first to outline the etiology, pathophysiology, and clinical presentation of what would later be named "Zenker's diverticulum". Notably, they advocated for non-surgical treatment options at the time [36]. Subsequently, in 1886, Wheeler performed the first successful resection of a Zenker's diverticulum, though the procedure was initially plagued by a high rate of early postoperative complications [37]. In 1909, Godmann suggested a two-stage surgical approach to mitigate these risks [3].

Lahey and Warren, in 1954, shared their extensive experience with this procedure, specifically performing diverticulopexy and mediastinal packing as the initial step, followed by diverticulum resection at a subsequent stage [38]. Earlier, in the 1940s, Harrington (1945) and Sweet (1947) had proposed a single-stage surgical solution, but their approach failed to adequately address issues related to cricopharyngeal muscle spasm, particularly in the upper esophageal sphincter [36]. To address this, Aubin introduced the concept of cricopharyngeal myotomy in combination with diverticulectomy in 1936. This technique was subsequently described by Payne and Clagett in 1965, yielding favorable outcomes [3].

In 1966, Ronald Belsey further refined these techniques by successfully combining diverticulopexy with cricopharyngeal myotomy [39]. Around the same time, endoscopic resection methods also began to gain traction, though they carried a notable risk of morbidity.

1.4 A Historical Overview of Gastroesophageal Reflux Disease

GERD, often recognized by the symptom of heartburn (pyrosis), has been documented for centuries, though its underlying mechanisms have only recently been understood. A key breakthrough occurred in 1956 when Fyke and Code, through manometric studies, identified the LES as a "high-pressure zone" [40]. This discovery shifted the focus of GERD treatment from external anatomical structures to intrinsic mechanisms, particularly the role of the LES in preventing reflux.

The concept of transdiaphragmatic hernias dates back to the 16th century, with notable descriptions from Ambroise Paré and Giovanni Battista Morgagni [3]. However, transhiatal hernias, where the stomach protrudes through the esophageal hiatus, were not fully recognized until the early 20th century, thanks to the development of contrast-enhanced radiography. The delay in understanding these hernias was likely due to limitations in autopsy techniques, which often overlooked the connection between the esophagus, diaphragm, and stomach [41].

In the 19th century, René Laënnec was the first to detect sounds associated with organs moving into the thorax through diaphragmatic defects. In 1853, Henry Ingersoll Bowditch reviewed 88 cases of diaphragmatic hernias reported between 1610 and 1846, identifying what were likely the first documented cases of paraesophageal hernias. Additionally, Charles Michel Billard described the first case of esophagitis in a child in 1828, and in 1855, Karl Rokitanski established the link between GERD and esophagitis [3].

In 1906, Wilder Tileston proposed that GERD was caused by cardiac insufficiency, offering a detailed description of esophagitis. Joseph Sheehan's introduction of direct esophagoscopy in 1920 allowed for visualization of esophageal lesions, facilitating a better understanding of peptic esophageal stenosis. The term "peptic esophagitis" first appeared in the English language medical literature, introduced by Asher Winkelstein [5].

1.4.1 The Development of GERD Surgical Treatments

Surgical treatments for GERD progressed in tandem with advancements in diagnostic methods. In 1919, Angelo Soresi described a pioneering abdominal procedure to repair hernias, involving the reduction of the hernia and repair of the diaphragmatic defect while preserving major structures like the esophagus and aorta [42]. In 1929, Stuart Harrington at the Mayo Clinic introduced a less invasive videothoracoscopic technique for severe hiatal hernias, which significantly reduced perioperative mortality and recurrence rates [43].

In 1926, Åke Akerlund coined the term "hiatal hernia" and classified them into three types: congenital hernias due to brachyesophagus, paraesophageal hernias, and axial hernias [44]. This classification helped surgeons choose the most appropriate interventions. With the identification of the LES in 1956, further refinements in GERD surgery followed. Phillip Allison and Norman Barrett made important contributions by linking GERD to hiatal hernia, ultimately leading to the development of modern antireflux surgery. Barrett also studied what became known as Barrett's esophagus, initially thought to be a congenital condition but later understood as a result of chronic acid exposure from GERD [45].

A major surgical advancement occurred in 1956 when Rudolf Nissen introduced the 360° gastric wrap, known as Nissen fundoplication, which became a key procedure in treating GERD [46]. Belsey also developed a notable technique that reduced the cardia into the abdomen and reshaped the His angle to strengthen the LES. His final version, the Belsey-Mark IV, achieved a five-year recurrence-free survival rate of 85% [47]. Surgeons like Lucius Hill and Mark Orringer further advanced hybrid surgical techniques, combining gastroplasty with Nissen fundoplication to treat complex GERD cases [48].

1.4.2 Minimally Invasive Advancements

In June 1989, laparoscopic antireflux surgery was pioneered by A. Cuschieri and his team in Dundee, employing the ligamentum teres cardiopexy technique previously described by Narbona-Arnau et al. [49]. The first documented laparoscopic Nissen fundoplication was performed in April 1991 by T. Geagea, a Lebanese surgeon working in Canada, using the Nissen-Rossetti modification [50]. Later that year, B. Dallemagne, a Belgian surgeon experienced in traditional antireflux surgery, also began performing laparoscopic Nissen fundoplications, which involved full mobilization of the gastric fundus by dividing the short gastric vessels [51].

Initial results from these pioneering groups were published in 1991. Geagea, in his report on ten cases, expressed optimism that the laparoscopic approach would lead to earlier referrals and prevent long-term complications associated with GERD [50]. Cuschieri's team reported favorable outcomes in eight elderly patients, noting quicker recovery times. Dallemagne's group, operating on twelve patients, utilized four laparoscopic ports for instrument insertion and completed a "floppy" 360° wrap with a nasogastric tube in place, followed by hiatal repair [51]. Their publication was influential in promoting the adoption of laparoscopic antireflux surgery, emphasizing the reduced need for large incisions, decreased postoperative pain, and faster recovery times.

These pioneering papers, much like Nissen's original work, are considered foundational in GERD surgery. After these initial reports, the global adoption of laparoscopic antireflux procedures surged, much like the trend with laparoscopic cholecystectomy. While this rapid uptake occurred without rigorous randomized controlled trials comparing laparoscopic methods to traditional open surgery, the procedure's comparable outcomes and minimally invasive nature led to its widespread acceptance among surgeons and patients alike [52]. Robotic surgery is currently considered a transformative advancement in the field of minimally invasive surgery. Since receiving clinical approval in 2000, robotic systems have become increasingly prevalent in general surgery [53]. Numerous studies have sought to evaluate the differences between conventional laparoscopic procedures and those assisted by robotic technology. In a study by J. Villamere et al., the use of robotic-assisted techniques in academic institutions was investigated. Their research, which compared robotic-assisted methods to traditional laparoscopy in common general surgical procedures, including antireflux surgery, found that robotics did not offer any additional benefits but was consistently associated with higher costs [54]. Similarly, M. Altieri et al. conducted a comparative analysis between laparoscopy and robotics in five major procedures, including esophageal fundoplication. Their findings showed no evidence of superior outcomes with the robotic approach for this procedure [55]. T. Gehrig et al. performed a retrospective analysis of 42 patients undergoing hiatal hernia repairs, comparing perioperative outcomes and hospital length of stay among 12 robotic, 17 laparoscopic, and 13 open surgeries [56]. Both minimally invasive techniques—robotic and laparoscopic—were shown to be safe alternatives to open surgery, with reduced hospital stays and fewer complications. However, when comparing robotic and laparoscopic approaches directly, no significant advantage of robotic surgery was observed regarding perioperative outcomes or length of stay [53]. Interestingly, the introduction of three-dimensional printing technology has recently revolutionized robotic surgery for GERD in complex cases. One notable advancement was introduced for the first time by Marano et al. in 2019, who conducted the first case of fundoplication using a 3D-printed model in combination with a robotic platform [57]. A 3D-printed model of the esophagus, thoracic aorta, and stomach was created based on computed tomography imaging, allowing precise preoperative planning and intraoperative guidance. Using the da Vinci Surgical System, surgeons were able to superimpose the 3D images onto the surgical field, facilitating a safer and more accurate dissection. This combination of 3D printing and robotics allowed for better orientation of critical structures, reducing operative risks and improving patient outcomes.

References

1. Aziz Q, Fass R, Gyawali CP, et al. Functional esophageal disorders. Gastroenterology. 2016;S0016-5085(16):00178–5.
2. Debas HT. Gastrointestinal Surgery. 1st ed. New York: Springer; 2004.
3. Brewer LA 3rd. History of surgery of the esophagus. Am J Surg. 1980;139(6):730–43.
4. Collis JL. The history of British oesophageal surgery. Thorax. 1982;37(11):795–802.
5. Deschamps C. History of esophageal surgery for benign disease. Chest Surg Clin N Am. 2000;10(1):135–44.
6. Olch PD. Johann von Mikulicz-Radecki. Ann Surg. 1960;152(5):923–6.
7. Robinson DH, Toledo AH. Historical development of modern anesthesia. J Invest Surg. 2012;25(3):141–9.
8. Bradley M, Nealiegh M, Oh JS, et al. Combat casualty care and lessons learned from the past 100 years of war. Curr Probl Surg. 2017;54(6):315–51.
9. Shemmeri E, Wee JO. Robotics and minimally invasive esophageal surgery. Ann Transl Med. 2021;9(10):898.
10. Thomas PA. Milestones in the history of esophagectomy: from Torek to minimally invasive approaches. Medicina (Kaunas). 2023;59(10):1786.
11. Willis T. Pharmaceutice rationalis. Sive Diatriba de medicamentorum operationibus in humano corpore. In Univ. Oxon. Prof. Sedleiano, nec non Coll. Med. Lond. & Societ. Reg. Socio. 1679.
12. Russel JC. Diagnosis and treatment of spasmodic stricture of the oesophagus. Br Med J. 1953;1898(1):1450–1.
13. Heller E, Heller K. Extramuskose cardioplastik beim Chronischen Cardiospasmus: Mit dilatation des oesophagus. Mitt Genzgeb. Med. Chir. 1913.
14. Mikulicz-Radecki J. Zur Pathologie und Therapie des Cardiospasmus. Deutsche Medizinische Wochenschrift. 1904.
15. Dor J, Humbert P, Paoli JM, et al. Treatment of reflux by the so-called modified Heller-Nissen technic. Presse Med (1893). 1967;75(50):2563–5.
16. Toupet A. Technic of esophago-gastroplasty with phrenogastropexy used in radical treatment of hiatal hernias as a supplement to Heller's operation in cardiospasms. Mem Acad Chir (Paris). 1963;89:384–9.
17. Cuschieri A. The spectrum of laparoscopic surgery. World J Surg. 1992;16(6):1089–97.
18. Pellegrini C, Wetter LA, Patti M, et al. Thoracoscopic esophagomyotomy. Initial experience with a new approach for the treatment of achalasia. Ann Surg. 1992;216(3):291–6.
19. Melvin WS, Needleman BJ, Krause KR, et al. Computer-assisted robotic heller myotomy: initial case report. J Laparoendosc Adv Surg Tech A. 2001;11(4):251–3.
20. Awshah S, Mhaskar R, Diab ARF, et al. Robotics vs laparoscopy in foregut surgery: systematic review and meta-analysis analyzing hiatal hernia repair and Heller myotomy. J Am Coll Surg. 2024;239(2):171–86.
21. Rake AT. Achalasia and degeneration of Auerbach's plexus. Proc R Soc Med. 1928;21(11):1775.
22. Hurst AF, Rake GW. Achalasia of the cardia: so-called cardiospasm. Q J Med. 1930;os-23(92):491–508.
23. Kronecker H, Meltzer SJ. Der Schluckmechanismus, seine Erregung und seine Hemmung. Arch Anat Physiol. 1883;7(Suppl):328–62.
24. Kramer P, Fleshler B, McNally E, Harris LD. Oesophageal sensitivity to Mecholyl in symptomatic diffuse spasm. Gut. 1967;8(2):120–7.
25. Clarke JO, Triadafilopoulos G. Esophageal motility disorders. Clin Gastrointestinal Endosc. 2019;220–233.e3.
26. Marano L, Pallabazzer G, Solito B, et al. Surgery or peroral esophageal myotomy for achalasia: a systematic review and meta-analysis. Medicine. 2016;95(10):e3001.

27. Di Martino N, Monaco L, Izzo G, et al. The effect of esophageal myotomy and myectomy on the lower esophageal sphincter pressure profile: intraoperative computerized manometry study. Dis Esophagus. 2005;18:160–5.
28. Pallabazzer G, Peluso C, de Bortoli N, et al. Clinical and pathophysiological outcomes of the robotic-assisted Heller-Dor myotomy for achalasia: a single-center experience. J Robot Surg. 2020;14(2):331–5.
29. Moonen A, Annese V, Belmans A, et al. Long-term results of the European achalasia trial: a multicentre randomised controlled trial comparing pneumatic dilation versus laparoscopic Heller myotomy. Gut. 2016;65(5):732–9.
30. Tuason J, Inoue H. Current status of achalasia management: a review on diagnosis and treatment. J Gastroenterol. 2017;52(4):401–6.
31. Del Genio A, Izzo G, Di Martino N, et al. Intraoperative esophageal manometry: our experience. Dis Esophagus. 1997;10(4):253–61.
32. Mattioli S, Pilotti V, Felice V, et al. Intraoperative study on the relationship between the lower esophageal sphincter pressure and the muscular components of the gastro-esophageal junction in achalasic patients. Ann Surg. 1993;218(5):635–9.
33. Stein HJ, Liebermann-Meffert D, DeMeester TR, Siewert JR. Three-dimensional pressure image and muscular structure of the human lower esophageal sphincter. Surgery. 1995;117(6):692–8.
34. Di Martino N, Marano L, Torelli F, et al. The calibrated laparoscopic Heller myotomy with fundoplication. Ann Ital Chir. 2013;84:19–24.
35. Virchow R. Handbuch der speciellen Pathologie und Therapie. Erlangen: Verlag von Ferdinand Enke; 1867.
36. Constantin A, Mates IN, Predescu D, et al. Principles of surgical treatment of Zenker diverticulum. J Med Life. 2012;5(1):92.
37. Wheeler D. Diverticula of the foregut. Radiology. 1947;49(4):476–82.
38. Lahey FH, Warren KW. Esophageal diverticula. Surg Gynecol Obstet. 1954;98(1):1–28.
39. Belsey R. Functional disease of the oesophagus. Postgrad Med J. 1963;39(451):290–8.
40. Code CF, Fyke FE, Schlegel JF. The gastroesophageal sphincter in healthy human beings. Gastroenterologia. 1956;86(3):135–50.
41. Franklin RH. Milestones in oesophageal surgery. J R Soc Med. 1971;64(3):257–60.
42. Soresi AL. Diaphragmatic hernia: its unsuspected frequency: its diagnosis: technic for radical cure. Ann Surg. 1919;69(3):254–70.
43. Harrington SW. Diaphragmatic hernia. Arch Surg. 1928;16(1):386–415.
44. Åkerlund ÅI. Hernia diaphragmatica hiatus oesophagei vom anatomischen und rontgenologischen gesichtspunkt. Acta Radiol. 1926;6(1–6):3–22.
45. Barrett NR. Hiatus hernia: a review of some controversial points. Br J Surg. 1954;42(173):231–44.
46. Nissen R. A simple operation for control of reflux esophagitis. Schweiz Med Wochenschr. 1956;86(Suppl 20):590–2.
47. Belsey R. Functional disease of the esophagus. J Thorac Cardiovasc Surg. 1966;52(2):164–88.
48. Orringer MB, Skinner DB, Belsey RH. Long-term results of the Mark IV operation for hiatal hernia and analyses of recurrences and their treatment. J Thorac Cardiovasc Surg. 1972;63(1):25–33.
49. Dávila DD. Profesor D. Benjamín Narbona Arnau. Rev Hispanoam Hernia. 2015;3:133–5.
50. Geagea T. Laparoscopic Nissen-Rossetti fundoplication. Surg Endosc. 1994;8(9):1080–4.
51. Dallemagne B, Weerts JM, Jeahes C, Markiewicz S. Results of laparoscopic Nissen fundoplication. Hepatogastroenterology. 1998;45(23):1338–43.
52. Anvari M. Outcomes of antireflux surgery. In: Swanstrom L, Dunst C, editors. Antireflux surgery. New York: Springer; 2014. p. 229–38.
53. Gonçalves-Costa D, Barbosa JP, Quesado R, et al. Robotic surgery versus laparoscopic surgery for anti-reflux and hiatal hernia surgery: a short-term outcomes and cost systematic literature review and meta-analysis. Langenbecks Arch Surg. 2024;409(1):175.

54. Villamere J, Gebhart A, Vu S, Nguyen NT. Utilization and outcome of laparoscopic versus robotic general and bariatric surgical procedures at Academic Medical Centers. Surg Endosc. 2015;29(7):1729–36.
55. Altieri MS, Yang J, Telem DA, et al. Robotic-assisted outcomes are not tied to surgeon volume and experience. Surg Endosc. 2016;30(7):2825–33.
56. Gehrig T, Mehrabi A, Fischer L, et al. Robotic-assisted paraesophageal hernia repair – a case-control study. Langenbecks Arch Surg. 2013;398(5):691–6.
57. Marano L, Ricci A, Savelli V, et al. From digital world to real life: a robotic approach to the esophagogastric junction with a 3D printed model. BMC Surg. 2019;19(1):153.

Open Access This chapter is licensed under the terms of the Creative Commons Attribution-NonCommercial 4.0 International License (http://creativecommons.org/licenses/by-nc/4.0/), which permits any noncommercial use, sharing, adaptation, distribution and reproduction in any medium or format, as long as you give appropriate credit to the original author(s) and the source, provide a link to the Creative Commons license and indicate if changes were made.

The images or other third party material in this chapter are included in the chapter's Creative Commons license, unless indicated otherwise in a credit line to the material. If material is not included in the chapter's Creative Commons license and your intended use is not permitted by statutory regulation or exceeds the permitted use, you will need to obtain permission directly from the copyright holder.

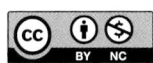

Esophageal Anatomy and Physiology. Epidemiology and Pathophysiology of Functional Disorders

2

Giovanni Aldinio, Beatrice Marinoni, Marina Coletta, and Roberto Penagini

2.1 Anatomy and Physiology of the Esophagus [1, 2]

The esophagus is a hollow, muscular tube located in the superior and posterior mediastinum, approximately 20–30 cm in length, that serves as a conduit between the pharynx and the stomach. It is bounded cranially by the upper esophageal sphincter (UES) and caudally by the lower esophageal sphincter (LES). The esophagus features a complex, multi-layered wall structure. The innermost layer is the mucosa, comprising a nonkeratinized stratified squamous epithelium, loose connective tissue (lamina propria), and a thin layer of smooth muscle (muscularis mucosae). Beneath this lies the submucosa, which consists of dense irregular connective tissue housing the neurons of the Meissner plexus and glands. The muscularis externa is organized into an inner circular and outer longitudinal muscle layer, with the neurons of the Auerbach plexus situated between them. The muscle fibers of the upper third of the esophagus and the UES are striated, transitioning to smooth muscle fibers from the proximal third up to the LES. Externally, the esophagus is covered by connective tissue (adventitia) in the cervical and thoracic regions for structural support, and by the visceral peritoneum (serosa) in the abdominal region.

G. Aldinio
University of Milan, Milan, Italy
e-mail: giovanni.aldinio95@gmail.com

B. Marinoni · M. Coletta
Fondazione IRCCS Ca' Granda Ospedale Maggiore Policlinico, Milan, Italy
e-mail: beatrice.marinoni@policlinico.mi.it; marina.coletta@policlinico.mi.it

R. Penagini (✉)
University of Milan, Milan, Italy

Fondazione IRCCS Ca' Granda Ospedale Maggiore Policlinico, Milan, Italy
e-mail: roberto.penagini@unimi.it

© The Author(s) 2026
V. Landolfi, S. Tolone (eds.), *Functional Diseases of the Esophagus*, Updates in Surgery, https://doi.org/10.1007/978-3-031-90570-4_2

The esophagus is innervated by the vagus nerve, which provides both somatic and visceral motor neurons. In healthy individuals, the innervation of the esophageal mucosa varies: nerve fibers are located deeper in the distal esophagus and nearer to the surface in the proximal esophagus.

Caudally, the esophagogastric junction (EGJ) works as a barrier between the esophagus and the stomach and is composed of the LES, the crural diaphragm, and a flap valve, formed by the phrenoesophageal ligament and the annular fibers of the gastric cardia.

2.1.1 Swallowing

Swallowing is a complex, multiphase process consisting of three main phases: the oral phase, the pharyngeal phase, and the esophageal phase. The oral phase involves mastication and bolus formation in the oral cavity. During the pharyngeal phase, coordination of several muscles pushes the bolus through the pharynx avoiding food being spread into the nose and into the airways. In the esophageal phase, both esophageal sphincters relax to allow passage of the bolus, while the esophageal body contracts in a coordinated manner to generate peristaltic waves (primary peristalsis) to propel food downward. Peristalsis can occur without swallowing, when it is triggered by esophageal distension induced by incomplete bolus clearance (secondary peristalsis).

Swallowing can be initiated voluntarily during eating and drinking or involuntarily when saliva or respiratory secretions accumulate in the pharynx. Swallowing is regulated by a network of neurons in the brainstem, known as the swallowing pattern generator (SPG), which coordinates the sequential and rhythmic motor activity required for swallowing. SPG activity is essential for airway protection, initiation of peristalsis, efficient bolus propulsion and coordination with other respiratory, cardiovascular, and gastrointestinal reflexes.

2.2 Gastroesophageal Reflux Disease [3–5]

Gastroesophageal reflux disease (GERD) is a condition in which retrograde flow of gastric contents causes troublesome symptoms, such as heartburn, regurgitation, and difficulty in swallowing, and/or complications, like erosive esophagitis, strictures, Barrett's esophagus and esophageal adenocarcinoma. In the U.S., approximately 110,000 annual hospital admissions occur as a result of GERD-related complications.

2.2.1 Epidemiology

GERD is a prevalent condition globally, with significant variation in occurrence across different regions. Accurately estimating GERD prevalence is challenging even within individual countries due to the variation in GERD definition among studies (based on symptoms and/or objective findings) and study methodologies. For instance, in the United States the estimated prevalence of GERD ranges from 6% to 30%, depending on the questionnaire used to assess the presence and severity of symptoms. The highest prevalence of GERD is observed in South Asia and Southeast Europe, where more than 25% of the population reports symptoms. In contrast, the prevalence is notably lower in Southeast Asia, Canada and France, where less than 10% of individuals report symptoms on a weekly basis. Notably, in the last 30 years, the prevalence of GERD symptoms in North America, Europe and Southeast Asia has risen by about 50%. However, due to the widespread use of proton pump inhibitors (PPIs), this increase has leveled off in recent years.

2.2.1.1 Risk Factors

Several risk factors for GERD have been identified, with variable degrees of strength of association.

In Western countries, no significant association between sex and the occurrence of GERD symptoms has yet been proven. In South America and the Middle East, however, women are about 40% more likely to experience and report symptoms of GERD compared to men. Conversely, men are at higher risk for complications of GERD. In the same way, the relationship between age and GERD symptoms has been variable, whereas a stronger correlation exists between older age and GERD complications.

Obesity is one of the most recognized risk factors for GERD: as body mass index (BMI) increases, the prevalence of GERD symptoms and erosive esophagitis rises. At the same time, engaging in moderate, consistent aerobic exercise has been proven as a protective factor against GERD symptoms. The use of tobacco and alcohol are also important risk factors for GERD and its complications. In particular, even if tobacco use is only weakly associated with GERD symptoms, it has a stronger association with erosive esophagitis and esophageal adenocarcinoma. Infection with *Helicobacter pylori*, especially the cytotoxin-associated gene A (Cag A) positive strains, has been found to be inversely related to GERD, erosive esophagitis, Barrett's esophagus, and esophageal adenocarcinoma. In the last 20 years, the decrease in incidence of *Helicobacter pylori* gastritis may also have been contributing to the increase of GERD.

2.2.2 Pathophysiology of Gastroesophageal Reflux Disease

The pathophysiology of GERD is multifactorial and complex, involving the interplay between anatomical structures such as the EGJ, physiological mechanisms like esophageal motility and clearance, and contributing factors including gastric contents, obesity and esophageal sensitivity.

2.2.2.1 Esophagogastric Junction

In GERD, the LES may be characterized by a lower basal pressure, resulting in a decrease of the sphincter tone and facilitating reflux. A decrease in LES pressure can be induced by factors such as increased intra-abdominal pressure, gastric distention and certain foods (e.g., carbonated beverages, chocolate) or medications (e.g., anticholinergic drugs, calcium-channel blockers). Physiological relaxations of the LES occur upon swallowing to allow food bolus passage, but also independently from it, a phenomenon known as "transient LES relaxation" (TLESR). These relaxations, lasting more than 10 seconds, predominantly occur during daytime postmeal periods and are triggered by a vagal reflex due to gastric distention. TLESRs have been shown to be the most common cause of gastroesophageal reflux in the presence of a normal LES pressure, both in patients with GERD symptoms and in asymptomatic individuals.

The presence of a hiatal hernia, occurring when part of the stomach passes into the thorax through an enlarged esophageal hiatus, increases the likelihood of reflux particularly when greater than 2 cm. Indeed, this anatomical defect impairs the ability of the EGJ to maintain the gastric contents in the stomach due to both changes of pressure dynamics around the LES and the LES misalignment with the crural diaphragm, especially during increased intra-abdominal pressure events such as deep inspiration or coughing.

2.2.2.2 Motility and Clearance

GERD patients may experience hypomotility affecting both primary and secondary peristalsis: ineffective esophageal motility is a common finding among GERD patients during high-resolution manometry. Actually, it is unclear which condition might cause the other: GERD could potentially cause reduced esophageal motility due to damage from acid reflux, or ineffective esophageal motility could predispose a person to GERD by impairing the clearance of refluxate from the esophagus. Additionally, some medications, such as anticholinergics, antidepressants and opioids, can also impair esophageal motility.

The residual acidity is cleared by saliva, which contains bicarbonate and epidermal growth factor, favoring mucosal healing. Thus, reduced salivation, present in conditions like connective tissue diseases, in the elderly and in individuals taking medications (e.g., anticholinergics and antidepressants), is associated with extended acid clearance times.

Lastly, abnormalities in gastric motility, such as an increased and prolonged post-prandial fundus relaxation (known as "accommodation"), have been documented to affect reflux volume. Notably, delayed gastric emptying is associated with a greater extent of reflux episodes reaching the upper esophagus, rather than an increase in total acid exposure.

2.2.2.3 Refluxate

Reflux episodes can differ depending on the composition of the refluxate and its pH level. The presence of bile acids in the refluxate and the extent of esophageal exposure to acid correlate with the severity of symptoms and mucosal damage. Symptoms are more likely when acid exposure is longer and more proximal and esophageal clearance is delayed. Gas reflux, known as belching, has also been associated with an increase of reflux.

Furthermore, a phenomenon known as the "acid pocket" can lead to short-segment acid reflux episodes. This occurs when, after meals, an area of unbuffered acidic gastric content located at the EGJ extends into the esophagus. Despite this being a physiological event, GERD patients show larger pockets than healthy controls.

2.2.2.4 Obesity

Obesity contributes to GERD by means of several mechanisms. In obese patients, the increased intra-abdominal pressure caused by visceral adipose tissue favors the formation of hiatal hernias and the occurrence of reflux episodes. Additionally, obesity alters hormone levels (i.e., leptin and ghrelin), leading to lower LES pressure and impaired gastrointestinal motility. High-calorie meals further delay gastric emptying and increase TLESRs, leading to more frequent reflux episodes.

Moreover, in bariatric surgery, sleeve gastrectomy tends to increase GERD symptoms and the prevalence of esophagitis, while Roux-en-Y gastric bypass usually reduces reflux events, highlighting the need to consider GERD when planning obesity treatments.

2.2.2.5 Esophageal Sensitivity

Symptom severity does not always match the acid exposure and extent of mucosal damage, reflecting the spectrum of different entities that where once included in GERD. Patients with non-erosive reflux disease (NERD) can experience symptoms as severe as those with esophagitis, and some may perceive physiological reflux as symptomatic due to esophageal hypersensitivity. Functional heartburn occurs in some patients without reflux or increased acid exposure. Differences among phenotypes may be explained by distinct mucosal nerve distributions. For example, patients with NERD have more superficial nerves, whereas conditions like Barrett's esophagus may lead to hyposensitivity, where severe lesions develop with mild or no symptoms.

Psychoneuroimmune factors can modulate esophageal sensitivity, with stress and sleep deprivation increasing sensitivity to acid. Reflux-induced inflammation sensitizes sensory nerves, and acute stress can cause changes in the esophageal mucosa that stimulate sensory nerves. Psychosocial factors, particularly esophageal hypervigilance, amplify GERD symptoms, creating a cycle of heightened awareness and symptom avoidance behaviors. This hypervigilance affects all GERD phenotypes and is a predictor of symptom severity, regardless of anxiety levels, potentially contributing to refractory GERD.

2.3 Esophageal Achalasia [6–12]

Achalasia is a rare neuromuscular disorder of the esophagus characterized by impaired relaxation of the LES and absent or spastic contractions in the esophageal body.

2.3.1 Epidemiology of Achalasia

The annual incidence of achalasia is estimated at 1–5 cases per 100,000 individuals with a prevalence of 7–32 cases per 100,000 individuals. Incidence is comparable across countries using similar epidemiological methodology and does not differ by ethnicity and gender. Achalasia can occur at any age, but the incidence and prevalence increase with age, and the mean age at diagnosis is >50 years.

2.3.2 Pathophysiology of Achalasia

The central pathophysiological abnormality in achalasia is the loss of inhibitory nerve function within the smooth muscle of the esophagus. In particular, nitric oxide-producing inhibitory neurons in the myenteric plexus, which are essential for the relaxation of esophageal smooth muscle, are primarily affected. In contrast, cholinergic neurons, which contribute to LES tone by inducing smooth muscle contraction, are relatively spared. The progressive neuro-inflammatory process causes the degeneration and subsequent loss of inhibitory ganglion cells within the myenteric plexus of the esophageal wall. In terms of neuronal dysfunction, achalasia type 1 and 2 are both characterized by loss of ganglion cells, with a gradient of more severe loss in type 1 achalasia, whereas in type 3 inhibitory neural function is impaired without clear neuronal loss. The different types of achalasia may be three distinct entities; however, some prospective data suggest the hypothesis that the different manometric patterns represent stages in the progression of the same disease, type 3 being the early one, type 2 the intermediate, and type 1 probably the end stage.

Autoimmunity is presently considered an important cause of the pathophysiological changes, leading to progressive degeneration of esophageal myenteric neurons, primarily through cell-mediated mechanisms with potential antibody-mediated processes in genetically predisposed individuals. Patients with achalasia not unfrequently present with autoimmune disorders, including Sjogren syndrome, type I diabetes mellitus and hypothyroidism, further supporting the hypothesis that achalasia has an autoimmune component.

Furthermore, viral DNA and virus-targeted antibodies have been found in esophageal tissue and in the serum, respectively, of patients with achalasia. Of particular interest is HSV-1, a neurotropic virus, suggesting the hypothesis that HSV-1 triggers immune activation.

The immune cells involved in the inflammatory process include eosinophils. Their degranulation releases toxic proteins capable of destroying myenteric neurons. A recent retrospective study using high resolution manometry (HRM) in a large cohort of patients showed that achalasia and obstructive motor disorders are found in 15% of patients with eosinophilic esophagitis, suggesting the relevance of esophageal eosinophilia in the development of these disorders.

Genetic predisposition also has a role in the pathogenesis since immunogenetic studies report an association between *HLA-DQw1*, *HLA-DQA1* and *HLA-DQB1*, and achalasia, with *HLA-DQB1* being the most commonly reported variant, especially in Southern Europe. Achalasia can be part of a genetic syndrome, i.e., the Allgrove syndrome (also termed AAA syndrome, which involves achalasia, alacrimia and adrenal insufficiency), from mutations on chromosome 12.

In patients with an HRM diagnosis of achalasia it is important to exclude the use of opioid drugs, not infrequently prescribed as analgesics. Opioids have been known for several years to interfere with esophageal inhibitory neural pathways, and chronic opioid use has been shown to cause the so-called opioid-induced esophageal dysfunction, a recently defined clinical syndrome characterized by esophageal symptoms and esophageal motility abnormalities, including achalasia type 3, hypercontractile esophagus, distal esophageal spasm, and esophagogastric junction outflow obstruction (EGJ-OO).

2.4 Hypercontractile Esophagus [13–16]

Hypercontractile esophagus (HE) is a primary disorder of peristalsis defined by an excessive peristaltic vigor (i.e., a distal contractile integral >8,000 mmHg·s·cm), which may include excessive LES after-contraction, not associated with a mechanical obstruction. HE, initially termed "nutcracker esophagus" in the era of conventional manometry, describes a disorder associated with non-cardiac chest pain or dysphagia and characterized by high amplitude, normally propagated peristaltic contractions.

2.4.1 Epidemiology of Hypercontractile Esophagus

HE is a rare disease. According to a meta-analysis including 38 case series of HE, the pooled prevalence of HE was 1.97% (95% CI: 1.39%–2.78%) among patients referred for HRM. The mean age at diagnosis was 60.8 years (95% CI: 57.1–64.4) and 65% (95% CI: 58%–72%) of patients were female.

2.4.2 Pathophysiology of Hypercontractile Esophagus

The primary pathophysiological mechanism underlying HE is thought to involve an excessive excitatory cholinergic drive within the myenteric plexus of the esophageal wall. This is associated with a temporal asynchrony between the circular and longitudinal muscle contractions of the esophagus, ultimately leading to exaggerated peristaltic contractions in the esophageal body. Although the exact etiological mechanism remains unclear and most cases are idiopathic, abnormal peripheral neural control and histopathological changes in the esophagus may play a significant role. Common histopathological findings in HE include the loss of inhibitory ganglion cells in the myenteric plexus and lymphocytic infiltration surrounding the ganglia, which are also characteristic of achalasia and EGJ-OO.

Although most cases are idiopathic, HE has been reported to occur in the context of EGJ mechanical obstruction, GERD, and opiate use. There is increasing evidence suggesting a link between HE and EGJ-OO. Several human and animal studies have shown that esophageal hypercontractility can be associated with impaired relaxation of the EGJ, indicating that HE may be a secondary phenomenon resulting from a distal obstructive process.

On the other hand, symptoms of GERD have been reported in approximately 40% of patients with HE and there is evidence that esophageal acid perfusion can induce multipeaked, repetitive, spontaneous, or simultaneous esophageal contractions. However, although the rate of symptom improvement with time is high in HE, it is independent of PPI use and/or the presence of GERD.

References

1. Rengarajan A, Gyawali CP. Functional anatomy and physiology of swallowing and esophageal motility. In: Richter JE, Castell DO, Katzka DA, Katz PO, Smout A, Spechler S, Vaezi MF, editors. The esophagus. 6th ed. Wiley; 2021. p. 59–96.
2. Pawlina W. Histology: a text and atlas: with correlated cell and molecular biology. 9th ed. Lippincott Williams & Wilkins, a Wolters Kluwer Business; 2024.
3. Richter JE, Rubenstein JH. Presentation and epidemiology of gastroesophageal reflux disease. Gastroenterology. 2018;154(2):267–76.
4. Arguero J, Sifrim D. Pathophysiology of gastro-oesophageal reflux disease: implications for diagnosis and management. Nat Rev Gastroenterol Hepatol. 2024;21(4):282–93.
5. Penagini R, Schoeman MN, Dent J, et al. Motor events underlying gastro-oesophageal reflux in ambulant patients with reflux oesophagitis. Neurogastroenterol Motil. 1996;8(2):131–41.
6. Harvey PR, Thomas T, Chandan JS, et al. Incidence, morbidity and mortality of patients with achalasia in England: findings from a study of nationwide hospital and primary care data. Gut. 2019;68(5):790–5.
7. Salvador R, Costantini M, Tolone S, et al. Manometric pattern progression in esophageal achalasia in the era of high-resolution manometry. Ann Transl Med. 2021;9(10):906.
8. Romero-Hernandez F, Furuzawa-Carballeda J, Hernandez-Molina G, et al. Autoimmune comorbidity in achalasia patients. J Gastroenterol Hepatol. 2018;33(1):203–8.
9. Castagliuolo I, Brun P, Costantini M, et al. Esophageal achalasia: is the herpes simplex virus really innocent? J Gastrointest Surg. 2004;8(1):24–30. discussion 30
10. Ghisa M, Laserra G, Marabotto E, et al. Achalasia and obstructive motor disorders are not uncommon in patients with eosinophilic esophagitis. Clin Gastroenterol Hepatol. 2021;19(8):1554–63.
11. Vackova Z, Niebisch S, Triantafyllou T, et al. First genotype-phenotype study reveals HLA-DQbeta1 insertion heterogeneity in high-resolution manometry achalasia subtypes. United Eur Gastroenterol J. 2019;7(1):45–51.
12. Snyder DL, Vela MF. Impact of opioids on esophageal motility. Neurogastroenterol Motil. 2023;35(5):e14587.
13. de Bortoli N, Gyawali PC, Roman S, et al. Hypercontractile esophagus from pathophysiology to management: proceedings of the Pisa Symposium. Am J Gastroenterol. 2021;116(2):263–73.
14. Wahba G, Bouin M. Jackhammer esophagus: a meta-analysis of patient demographics, disease presentation, high-resolution manometry data, and treatment outcomes. Neurogastroenterol Motil. 2020;32(11):e13870.

15. Mauro A, Quader F, Tolone S, et al. Provocative testing in patients with jackhammer esophagus: evidence for altered neural control. Am J Physiol Gastrointest Liver Physiol. 2019;316:G397–403.
16. Mallet AL, Ropert A, Bouguen G, et al. Prevalence and characteristics of acid gastro-oesophageal reflux disease in jackhammer oesophagus. Dig Liver Dis. 2016;48(10):1136–41.

Open Access This chapter is licensed under the terms of the Creative Commons Attribution-NonCommercial 4.0 International License (http://creativecommons.org/licenses/by-nc/4.0/), which permits any noncommercial use, sharing, adaptation, distribution and reproduction in any medium or format, as long as you give appropriate credit to the original author(s) and the source, provide a link to the Creative Commons license and indicate if changes were made.

The images or other third party material in this chapter are included in the chapter's Creative Commons license, unless indicated otherwise in a credit line to the material. If material is not included in the chapter's Creative Commons license and your intended use is not permitted by statutory regulation or exceeds the permitted use, you will need to obtain permission directly from the copyright holder.

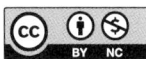

Radiological Evaluation of Functional Diseases of the Esophagus

3

Alfonso Reginelli, Vittorio Patanè, and Roberto Grassi

3.1 Normal Esophageal Function and Lower Esophageal Sphincter: Primary and Secondary Peristalsis

In 95–96% of patients, swallowing a bolus causes a main peristaltic wave of contraction that moves at a speed of 2–3.5 cm/s. According to manometric research, the lower esophageal sphincter maintains a resting basal pressure and relaxes a few seconds after the swallow is started. Radiologically, as the bolus reaches the gastroesophageal junction, it forces open the sphincter. The sphincter contracts once more as soon as the bolus passes, closing to preserve its barrier function. Any leftover food in the esophagus or the occurrence of gastroesophageal reflux may cause a subsequent peristaltic wave.

3.1.1 Non-propulsive Peristalsis

Non-propulsive contractions can be seen in the esophagus during videofluoroscopy or manometry (Fig. 3.1). Non-peristaltic waves can be assessed on conventional radiography as small irregularities along the lateral contour of the esophageal lumen, visible after the oral administration of a barium contrast medium.

3.1.2 Radiological Assessment of Esophageal Motility

The esophageal body, upper esophageal sphincter, and lower esophageal sphincter are always evaluated in radiological assessments of esophageal function. Studies

---

A. Reginelli (✉) · V. Patanè · R. Grassi
Department of Precision Medicine, University of Campania "Luigi Vanvitelli", Naples, Italy
e-mail: alfonso.reginelli@unicampania.it; vittorio.patane@unicampania.it; roberto.grassi@unicampania.it

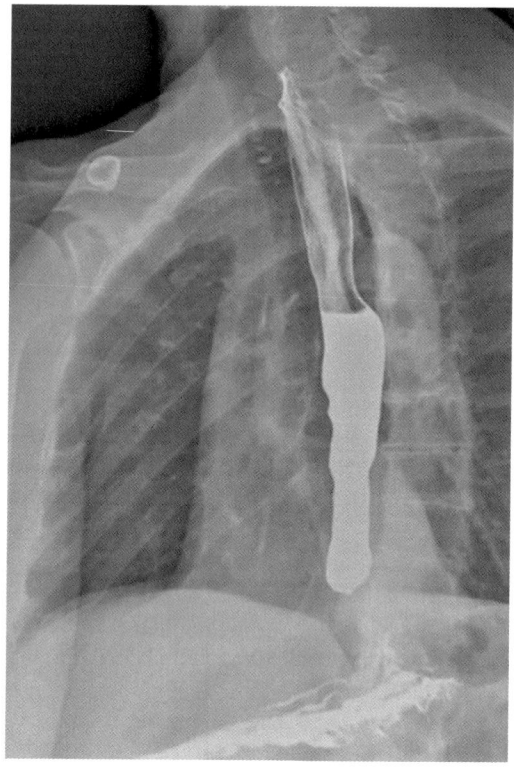

Fig. 3.1 X-ray performed in left anterior oblique projection after barium swallow. The lateral profile of the esophagus shows some irregularities, likely due to non-propulsive peristalsis

evaluating esophageal motor function should use low-density barium (about 100% weight by volume), and are carried out with the patient in an upright position. After a barium swallow, the esophageal lumen is occluded by the peristaltic contraction wave, giving the bolus tail its distinctive inverted "V" shape. The entire bolus is successfully propelled past the esophagus and into the stomach by this wave. In the upright position, bolus transit through the esophagus is usually quick. A persisting air-fluid level (sometimes referred to as a "support level") may be indicative of a stenosis or a motility problem.

3.2 Examination Technique

The patient is instructed to take a single swallow of a low-density barium bolus while in an upright left posterior oblique (LPO) position. The LPO position enables a better view of the gastroesophageal junction as it reduces the overlap between the esophagus and the spine. When assessing for gastroesophageal reflux, this can be generated by provocative testing or it can occur naturally during the examination. A solid bolus may be utilized for additional assessment if a patient has dysphagia for solids and the liquid barium examination is unable to identify the cause. There is currently no established reference value for evaluating solid transit time, and some individuals may have sluggish transit times for solid food. The mucosal lining is evaluated radiologically with a double-contrast examination of the esophagus.

3.2.1 Timed Barium Esophagogram

With a few adjustments, the timed barium esophagogram (TBE) technique is comparable to the standard barium swallow (Fig. 3.2). For example, it involves taking several consecutive films at predetermined intervals following a single swallow of a specified volume of a barium suspension with a particular density. It is recommended that patients fast overnight before TBE. The entire study is conducted in an upright position. Within 15 to 20 seconds, a low density barium sulfate suspension (45% weight by volume) is taken orally. The amount of suspension administered is often 100–250 mL, which should be sufficient to fill a dilated achalasic esophagus and be well tolerated by the patient without regurgitation or aspiration. As a standard protocol, a predetermined volume is preferable. LPO views are then obtained one, two, and five minutes after barium administration.

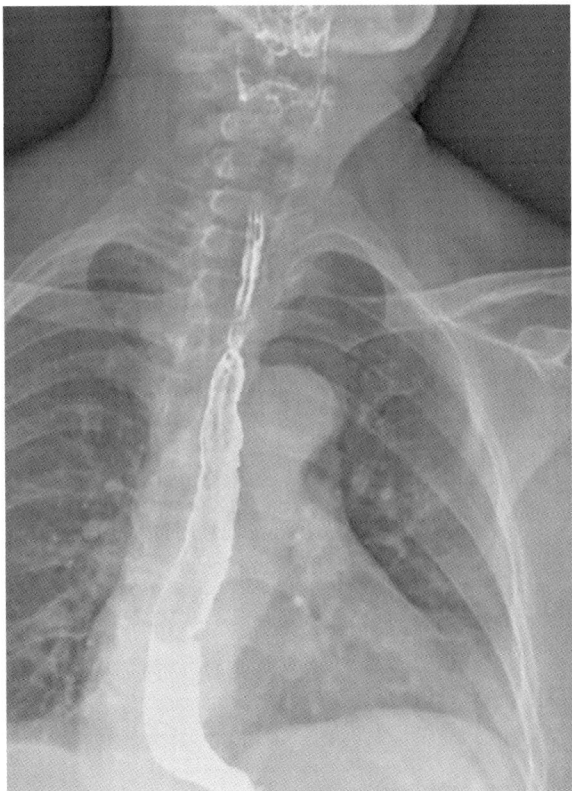

Fig. 3.2 Timed barium esophagogram obtained 1 min after barium contrast administration showing minimal dilatation of the esophageal lumen and retention of contrast medium within the esophagus, with appearance of a contrast-air level at the cranial end of the barium column

3.3 Esophageal Motility Disorders

Esophageal motility disorders are categorized using the most recent Chicago Classification (version 4). A wide variety of motor abnormalities occurring in association with other diseases are known as secondary motility disorders. Detection of a known extraesophageal condition is also necessary for the identification of a secondary motility disorder. The best course of treatment depends on detailed knowledge of the specific manometric abnormality, and can vary greatly. Esophageal motility abnormalities can be consistently detected and characterized with radiographic assessment.

3.4 Primary Motility Disorders

3.4.1 Achalasia

With an annual incidence of 1 case per 100,000 people and a prevalence of 10 cases per 100,000, achalasia is the most well-known esophageal motility disorder. The primary radiological sign is insufficient relaxation of the lower esophageal sphincter's, which is associated with aperistalsis in the esophageal body and the sphincter's inability to open during swallowing. Esophageal dilatation and a beak-like constriction of the lower esophageal sphincter are commonly seen on videofluoroscopy (Fig. 3.3). The esophagus may have a normal diameter in the early stages but, as the condition progresses, it dilates and retains food and saliva, eventually developing into an advanced form that gives the esophagus a "sock-like" appearance.

The sensitivity of the barium swallow in identifying achalasia varies from 58% to 95% since esophageal morphological abnormalities only become apparent in more advanced cases.

3.4.2 Diffuse Esophageal Spasm

Diffuse esophageal spasm occurs less frequently than achalasia. The presence of intense non-propulsive contractions, which can result in an esophageal curvature or a "corkscrew" appearance—also known as a "rosary bead" pattern—is one of the typical radiological signs of diffuse spasm (Fig. 3.4). A definite diagnosis of diffuse esophageal spasm cannot be made owing to the frequently vague radiological findings. Therefore, manometry is recommended for all individuals displaying radiographic evidence of a non-specific esophageal contractile abnormality and unexplained chest discomfort.

Fig. 3.3 X-ray performed in anteroposterior projection shows dilatation of the cervical esophagus with a progressive reduction in diameter towards the cardiac region, where an initial threadlike narrowing of the cardia can be seen. Subsequent manometric evaluation in this patient revealed dynamic-functional alterations consistent with achalasia

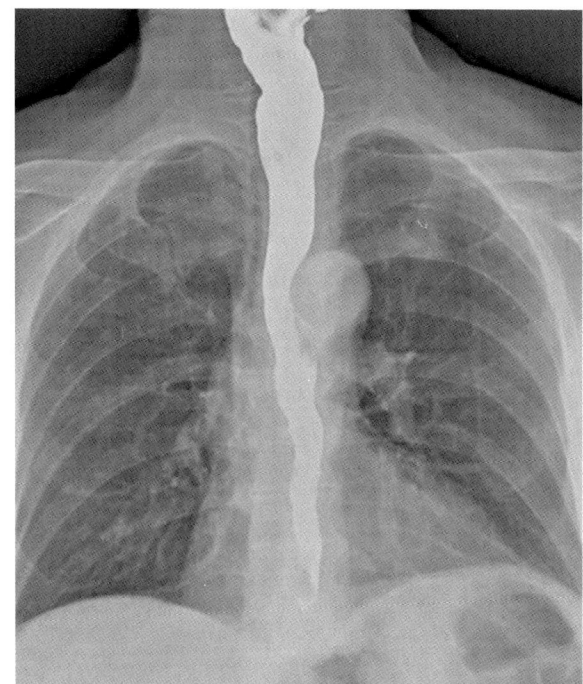

Fig. 3.4 X-ray performed in left anterior oblique projection after enteral administration of a barium contrast agent shows alternating stenotic segments and segments of normal caliber. Progression of the contrast agent is delayed, as evidenced by the areas of stasis. The image is consistent with an esophageal motility dysfunction suggestive of diffuse esophageal spasm

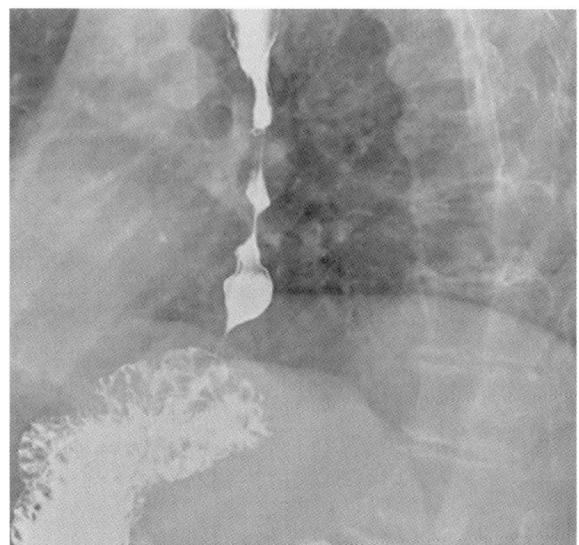

3.4.3 Nutcracker Esophagus

A nutcracker esophagus maintains primary peristalsis, but prolonged high-amplitude contractions can result in chest discomfort and dysphagia. Despite being crucial for the diagnosis, manometric examination is often not the first diagnostic method used in patients complaining of non-cardiac chest discomfort.

The persistence of peristaltic movements makes the radiographic diagnosis of nutcracker esophagus difficult. Overall, little is known about the pathophysiology of nutcracker esophagus. More research is needed to clarify the precise mechanisms at work, even though some data suggest that the condition may progress to achalasia, pointing to the existence of a potential spectrum of esophageal motility disorders.

3.4.4 Other Primary Esophageal Motility Disorders

Non-specific contractile abnormalities are the most prevalent group of esophageal motility disorders. A number of extraesophageal diseases may have these conditions as their primary or secondary cause. Multiple-peak contraction waves, peristaltic waves with diminished amplitude, and isolated simultaneous or spontaneous contractions can all be seen on manometry. Radiographic studies have a sensitivity of only 46–73% because contractility irregularities might be detected infrequently. Investigating the underlying conditions that can cause esophageal motility dysfunction (secondary motor disorders), such as diabetes, alcoholism, eosinophilic esophagitis, or progressive systemic sclerosis, is crucial from a clinical point of view.

3.4.5 Presbyesophagus

When Soergel et al. discovered that a significant number of older subjects had esophageal motility abnormalities, they coined the term "presbyesophagus". Ten out of fifteen individuals in their study of nonagenarians had non-propulsive contractions. It has been proposed that the increasing frequency of conditions such as diabetes and neuromuscular disorders, which can affect esophageal motility, probably underlies the increased prevalence of esophageal motility abnormalities. It has recently been shown that as people age, their esophageal transit times for liquid boluses increase noticeably. However, before establishing a diagnosis of a motility disorder in older adults with recent onset of dysphagia, it is important to rule out the presence of a tumor or stenosis.

3.4.6 Secondary Esophageal Motility Disorders

Esophageal dysmotility is a well-known characteristic of progressive systemic sclerosis (also known as scleroderma) and other connective tissue disorders. A dilated lower esophageal sphincter and the lack of peristalsis are two signs of hypomotility of the distal esophagus caused by esophageal involvement in progressive systemic sclerosis, which affects the smooth musculature.

On radiography, the esophagus may appear air-distended for a considerable amount of time after a swallow, without exhibiting the usual luminal collapse brought on by a peristaltic contraction. The distal esophagus shows hypomotility and barium retention on prone oblique views. With disease progression, a dilated lower esophageal sphincter and esophageal dilatation become evident. Complete aperistalsis and significant barium retention will be seen in the prone oblique position.

3.4.7 Diabetes Mellitus

Patients affected by diabetes frequently experience esophageal symptoms, and their risk of developing dysphagia is more than three times greater than that of non-diabetic controls. Weak peristalsis and an increased frequency of non-propulsive contractions are signs of esophageal motility failure. In diabetic patients, esophageal dysmotility is far more common than gastroparesis. Weak peristalsis or non-propulsive contractions may be seen on radiography.

3.4.8 Chagas Disease

Trypanosoma cruzi infection is the cause of Chagas disease, also known as South American trypanosomiasis. Cardiomegaly, megaesophagus, and megacolon are the most common features of the chronic phase of the disease, which primarily affects the heart, esophagus, and colon.

Chagas disease and achalasia might have the same radiological and clinical presentation. The correct diagnosis may also be inferred from the patient's place of origin, and serological testing is required to confirm a diagnosis of Chagas disease.

3.4.9 Motility Disorder-Related Esophageal Diverticula

Because esophageal diverticula (Fig. 3.5) are typically linked to an esophageal motility disorder, they have been included in this chapter. Location of the diverticulum will determine its classification: a mid-esophageal diverticulum is located just below the level of the aortic arch, an epiphrenic diverticulum is located just above the diaphragm, and a Zenker diverticulum is located above the pharyngoesophageal sphincter. Mid-esophageal diverticula were once generally regarded as traction diverticula of no therapeutic importance. Numerous more recent investigations have cast doubt on this theory, demonstrating that these diverticula more closely resemble pulsion diverticula. The underlying esophageal motility failure typically linked to epiphrenic diverticula is probably a contributing cause.

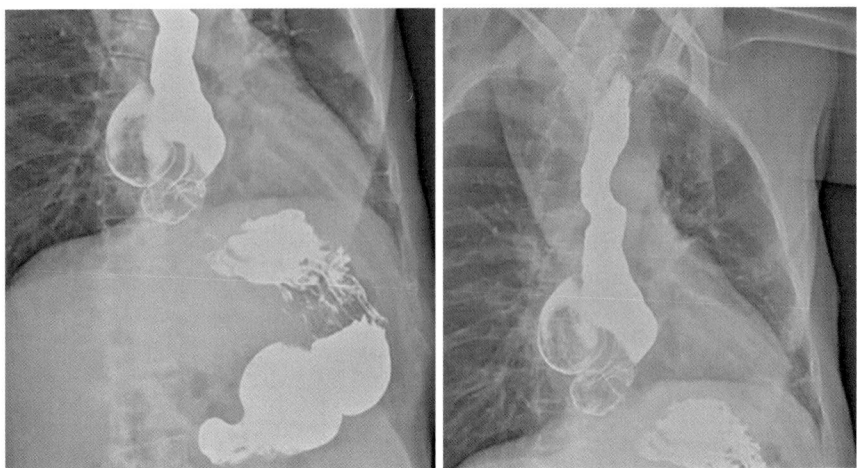

Fig. 3.5 Delayed progression of contrast agent in the esophagus. Dilatation of the esophageal lumen with a maximum diameter of approximately 45 mm. Evidence of a diverticulum on the right esophageal wall in the interbronchial region, with a neck of about 28 mm and a diameter of 63 mm, with contrast agent retention. Post-operative evidence of fundoplication according to Heller-Dor. Normally located stomach, patent pylorus, and normal morphology of the duodenal bulb and C-loop

3.5 Gastroesophageal Reflux Disease and Esophageal Motility

The whole range of esophageal histological alterations and clinical symptoms caused by gastroesophageal reflux are referred to as gastroesophageal reflux disease, or GERD. In the general population, GERD is by far the most frequent cause of esophagitis. Anatomical distortions of the gastroesophageal junction, including but not limited to hiatal hernia, or temporary relaxations of the lower esophageal sphincter without anatomical abnormalities are the main mechanisms that have been identified recently.

Suggested Reading

Aziz Q, Fass R, Gyawali CP, et al. Functional esophageal disorders. Gastroenterology. 2016;S0016–5085(16):00178–5.

Buchanan ME, Fishman EK, Azadi JR. CT evaluation of the esophagus: the role of CT imaging and CT imaging findings in diagnosing esophageal abnormalities. Curr Probl Diagn Radiol. 2023;52(4):289–99.

Grishaw EK, Ott DJ, Frederick MG, et al. Functional abnormalities of the esophagus: a prospective analysis of radiographic findings relative to age and symptoms. AJR Am J Roentgenol. 1996;167(3):719–23.

Summerton SL. Radiographic evaluation of esophageal function. Gastrointest Endosc Clin N Am. 2005;15(2):231–42.

Open Access This chapter is licensed under the terms of the Creative Commons Attribution-NonCommercial 4.0 International License (http://creativecommons.org/licenses/by-nc/4.0/), which permits any noncommercial use, sharing, adaptation, distribution and reproduction in any medium or format, as long as you give appropriate credit to the original author(s) and the source, provide a link to the Creative Commons license and indicate if changes were made.

The images or other third party material in this chapter are included in the chapter's Creative Commons license, unless indicated otherwise in a credit line to the material. If material is not included in the chapter's Creative Commons license and your intended use is not permitted by statutory regulation or exceeds the permitted use, you will need to obtain permission directly from the copyright holder.

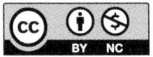

Functional Motor Disorders of the Esophagus

4

Nicola de Bortoli and Irene Solinas

4.1 Introduction

Patients presenting with esophageal symptoms such as dysphagia or chest pain potentially are affected by esophageal motor disorders. Those symptoms represent the first complaint and the most common reasons for referral to a gastroenterologist. The role of esophageal manometry in clinical practice includes accurately assessing esophageal motor function, identifying motor dysfunction, and guiding treatment plans based on these abnormalities.

This chapter provides a brief overview of the major esophageal motor disorders.

Esophageal high-resolution manometry (HRM) is considered the gold standard for diagnosing esophageal motor disorders. It utilizes color pressure topography, revolutionizing the classification of motor abnormalities through a hierarchical system known as the Chicago Classification. The first version of this classification was introduced in 2009, with the latest revision (version 4.0) released in January 2021 by the International HRM Working Group [1].

Esophageal motor disorders can stem from dysfunction in various areas: the upper esophageal sphincter (UES) and/or the cervical esophagus, which contain striated muscle (the proximal 3–5 cm); the mid and distal esophagus, which consist of smooth muscle; and the lower esophageal sphincter (LES) or esophagogastric junction (EGJ), where the LES interacts with the crural diaphragm (CD) to regulate function.

Disorders of the UES typically arise from abnormalities in the striated muscle or the extrinsic neurological system. These disorders often result in oropharyngeal dysphagia, which may be caused by improper relaxation of the UES or the tongue base region. The primary causes of oropharyngeal dysphagia include:

N. de Bortoli (✉) · I. Solinas
Division of Gastroenterology, Department of Translational Research and New Technologies in Medicine and Surgery, University of Pisa, Pisa, Italy
e-mail: nicola.debortoli@unipi.it; irenesolinas00@gmail.com

1. Central nervous system diseases (e.g., Parkinson's disease, transient ischemic attack or stroke, amyotrophic lateral sclerosis, Huntington's disease)
2. Cranial nerve disorders (e.g., recurrent laryngeal nerve paralysis, diphtheria, lead poisoning)
3. Skeletal muscle disorders (e.g., inflammatory myopathies, polymyositis, myasthenia gravis, myotonic dystrophy, muscular dystrophy).

Esophageal motor function and bolus transit can be assessed through various tests, including barium X-rays, scintigraphy, and more recently, intraluminal impedance. HRM is now widely regarded as the gold standard for evaluating esophageal motor activity.

Solid-state esophageal HRM is equipped with numerous pressure sensors (up to 36) that are spaced closely together. Compared to conventional manometry, HRM offers several advantages: it eliminates the need for a pull-through technique to detect the sphincters, and positional shifts do not compromise the accuracy or consistency of pressure readings. Additionally, data visualization has been enhanced by interpolation between sensors, enabling the display of esophageal pressure topography as seamless, color-coded isobaric regions representing esophageal motility and sphincter function. Both the UES and LES are clearly visible as high-pressure zones.

Before the procedure, patients are required to fast for at least 6 hours for solids and 2 hours for liquids. The test involves a brief observation of the resting EGJ, followed by the recording of motor activity during 10 swallows of 5 mL of water, each spaced 30 seconds apart. This standard protocol was recently updated in Chicago Classification version 4.0 [1]. The detailed protocol for esophageal HRM, as outlined in Chicago Classification version 4.0, can be found in Table 4.1. Any medications that may affect esophageal motility should be discontinued a few days prior to the test, if possible.

Table 4.1 Standard protocol for esophageal high-resolution manometry according to the Chicago Classification 4.0 [1]

Supine position	
Resting pressure	A baseline period of at least 30 seconds is captured to enable identification of anatomic landmarks including the UES and LES.
Esophageal peristalsis evaluation	Ten 5-mL wet swallows with water or saline (when using impedance) spaced 20–30 seconds apart.
Multiple rapid swallows	Five 2-mL wet swallows 2 seconds apart (within 10 s).
Secondary (upright) position	
Resting pressure	A baseline period of at least 30 seconds is captured to enable identification of anatomic landmarks including the UES and LES.
Upright peristalsis evaluation	Five 5-mL wet swallows with water or saline (when using impedance) spaced 20–30 seconds apart. In an upright position the IRP value of the LES/EGJ is normal when <12 mmHg.
Rapid drinking challenge (200 mL)	200 mL water, ingested as fast as possible through a straw

EGJ esophagogastric junction, *IRP* integrated relaxation pressure, *LES* lower esophageal sphincter, *UES* upper esophageal sphincter

4.1.1 Esophagogastric Junction Morphology

The EGJ consists of two main structures: the LES and the CD. EGJ morphology is categorized into three distinct types: *Type I*, where CD and LES completely overlap with no separation visible on the Clouse plot; *Type II*, where LES and CD are partially separated, producing a double-peaked spatial pressure plot, though the pressure between peaks remains above gastric levels; and *Type III*, where LES and CD are clearly separated, forming a double-peaked pressure plot with the nadir pressure at or below gastric pressure. Different EGJ characteristics—such as type, resting pressure, and contractile integral—have shown correlations with gastroesophageal reflux disease (GERD) [2].

During swallowing, EGJ relaxation is assessed through integrated relaxation pressure (IRP), calculated as the average of the 4 seconds (contiguous or non-contiguous) of maximal deglutitive relaxation within a 10-second window starting at UES relaxation. Using a 4-second IRP cutoff of 15 mmHg achieves optimal detection of achalasia, with 98% sensitivity and 96% specificity.

4.1.2 Esophageal Pressure Topography Metrics for Evaluating Swallows

The primary HRM metrics used to assess esophageal contractile function during swallowing are the distal contractile integral (DCI) and distal latency (DL). The DCI quantifies the strength of the esophageal contraction, measuring amplitude, duration, and length (in mmHg·s·cm) within the distal esophagus, using a 20 mmHg isobaric contour from proximal to distal pressure troughs. This metric was introduced as part of the Chicago Classification. Meanwhile, the DL measures the time between UES relaxation and the deceleration point along the 30 mmHg isobaric contour, marking where the propagation speed decreases and distinguishing the tubular esophagus from the phrenic ampulla. This point is known as the contractile deceleration point (CDP). DL offers an indirect assessment of deglutitive inhibition and normal peristalsis, with values below 4.5 seconds indicating a premature contraction (Fig. 4.1). Details on peristaltic wave characteristics, including contraction vigor and pattern, are summarized in Table 4.2.

The following sections of this chapter focus on the primary esophageal motor disorders identified through HRM. The current classification of these disorders is outlined in the Chicago Classification version 4.0 (2021) (Table 4.3). The classification's initial version was established in 2009 after an international gastroenterology conference, Digestive Disease Week, held in San Diego in May 2008. The second version was developed in 2012 following the International High Resolution Manometry Working Group meeting in Ascona, Switzerland, in April 2011. The latest version was compiled through virtual meetings held throughout 2020 during the global COVID-19 lockdown.

Fig. 4.1 Metrics of high-resolution manometry (HRM). Two high pressure zones are present: upper and lower esophageal sphincters (the latter included into the esophagogastric junction). The white squared area refers to distal contractile integral (DCI) calculation by means of 20 mmHg isobaric contour. The contractile deceleration point (CDP) is easily identifiable; it allows the calculation of distal latency (DL)

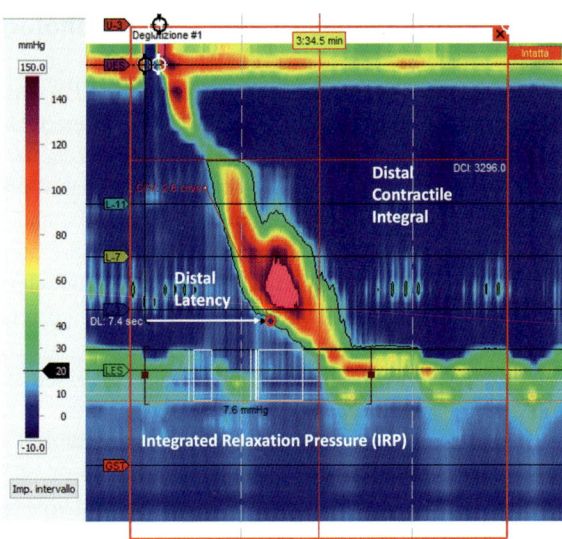

Table 4.2 Metrics of high-resolution manometry

Parameter	Definition	Values
IRP	Mean/median of the 4 seconds of maximal deglutitive relaxation in the 10-second window beginning at UES relaxation.	<15 mmHg (normal) >15 mmHg (abnormal)
DCI	Represents the vigor of contraction: amplitude x duration x length (mmHg·s·cm) of the distal esophageal contraction exceeding 20 mmHg from the transition zone to the proximal margin of the LES.	<100 failed 100–450 weak 450–8000 normal >8000 hypercontractile
DL	Interval between UES relaxation and the CDP (normal value 4.5 s). It represents the esophageal relaxation that precedes the contractile wave.	>4.5 s normal <4.5 s premature
CDP	Inflection point along the 30 mmHg isobaric contour at which propagation velocity slows demarcating the tubular esophagus from the phrenic ampulla.	
Panesophageal pressurization	Uniform pressurization extending from the UES to the EGJ with 30 mmHg isobaric contour.	
Fragmented wave	A peristaltic wave (DCI >450) with a large break (>5 cm) along the 20 mmHg isobaric contour.	

CDP contractile deceleration point, *DCI* distal contractile integral, *DL* distal latency, *EGJ* esophagogastric junction, *IRP* integrated relaxation pressure, *LES* lower esophageal sphincter, *UES* upper esophageal sphincter

Table 4.3 The Chicago Classification of esophageal motor disorders. Version 4.0

IRP > 15 mmHg	Disorders of the EGJ
Achalasia type 1	100% failed contractions
Achalasia type 2	100% failed contractions with panesophageal pressurization occurring with at least 20% of swallows
Achalasia type 3	No normal peristalsis; there is some residual motor activity in the distal esophagus with at least 20% premature contractions, defined as a DL <4.5 seconds.
EGJ-OO	A manometric diagnosis of EGJ-OO is always considered clinically inconclusive. It is defined as an elevated median IRP in the primary (IRP <15 mmHg) and secondary position (IRP >12 mmHg) and $\geq$ 20% swallows with elevated intrabolus pressure in the supine position, with evidence of peristalsis. Conclusive diagnosis of EGJ-OO requires clinically relevant symptoms with supportive investigations supporting obstruction (TBE).
IRP < 15 mmHg	**Disorders of peristalsis**
Aperistalsis	100% of failed contractions (DCI <100 mmHg·s·cm).
Distal esophageal spasm	100% normal contractions with at least 20% or more premature contractions defined as a DL < 4.5 s.
Hypercontractile esophagus	Normal peristalsis with occurrence of $\geq$20% of swallows with a DCI >8000 mmHg·s·cm and normal latency.
Ineffective esophageal motility	50% or more failed peristalsis (DCI <100 mmHg·s·cm). More than 70% ineffective swallows. Ineffective swallows may be failed or weak (DCI 100–450 mmHg·s·cm). More than 70% fragmented waves (DCI >450 mmHg·s·cm) with large break (>5 cm).
	Normal
Normal	Not achieving any of the above diagnostic criteria.

DCI distal contractile integral, *DL* distal latency, *EGJ* esophagogastric junction, *EGJ-OO* esophagogastric junction outflow obstruction, *IRP* integrated relaxation pressure, *TBE* timed barium esophagogram

4.1.3 Esophageal Pressure Topography Metrics for Scoring Individual Swallows

HRM peristaltic metrics commonly employed to assess esophageal contractile function include DCI and DL. The DCI measures the contractile strength of esophageal peristalsis, introduced within the framework of the Chicago Classification. It quantifies the amplitude, duration, and length (expressed in mmHg·s·cm) of distal esophageal contraction, calculated along a 20 mmHg isobaric contour from proximal to distal troughs. DL measures the interval from the onset of UES relaxation to the point along the 30 mmHg isobaric contour where propagation velocity slows, marking the transition from the tubular esophagus to the phrenic ampulla, also known as the CDP. DL indirectly evaluates deglutitive inhibition and normal peristalsis, with values below 4.5 seconds indicating premature contraction. Peristaltic wave characteristics, such as contractile vigor and pattern, are detailed in Table 4.1.

The following sections of this chapter discuss major esophageal motility disorders identified through HRM, based on the latest Chicago Classification version 4.0 (2021) [3].

4.2 Disorders of the Esophagogastric Junction

4.2.1 Esophageal Achalasia

Definition: Achalasia is characterized by an esophageal outflow obstruction resulting from abnormal relaxation of the LES due to defective inhibitory control, alongside impaired esophageal peristalsis.

Epidemiology: Achalasia has an annual incidence of 1 in 100,000 individuals and a prevalence of 10 in 100,000. It shows no significant racial or gender predilection, with symptom onset possible at any age but most frequently occurring between 30 and 60 years.

Etiology: Achalasia is generally an idiopathic condition with unknown causes, although a minority of cases in South America are attributed to *Trypanosoma cruzi* infection (Chagas disease). The disorder results from neuronal degeneration in the esophageal wall, with histology revealing a reduced number of ganglion cells in the myenteric plexuses. Degeneration primarily affects nitric oxide-producing inhibitory neurons, which facilitate the relaxation of esophageal smooth muscle, while cholinergic neurons that contribute to LES tone via smooth muscle contraction are often relatively preserved. This neuronal degeneration may stem from a T lymphocyte-mediated immune response, potentially influenced by genetic factors (such as HLA locus predispositions), and viral infections have also been suggested as a possible trigger.

The disordered motility characteristic of achalasia is largely due to a loss of inhibitory neurons in the esophageal wall. In the LES, this loss of inhibitory innervation leads to increased basal sphincter pressure, preventing normal relaxation. In the esophageal smooth muscle, it results in aperistalsis.

Clinical presentation: The primary symptom is dysphagia, affecting both solids and liquids in approximately 90% of patients, which may initially be intermittent or continuous. Patients often adapt by eating more slowly and may describe themselves as "slow eaters". Unlike dysphagia caused by structural obstructions, achalasia-related dysphagia is commonly accompanied by regurgitation of undigested food or saliva, which can occur even hours after a meal. This regurgitation, reported in 60–70% of patients, often lacks the acidic taste associated with reflux-related regurgitation. Some patients may experience aspiration pneumonia (*ab ingestis pneumonitis*) due to regurgitation. Occasionally, patients report chest pain or heartburn (in fewer than 30% of cases), which should be differentiated from GERD. Significant weight loss is usually a late symptom.

Diagnosis: HRM is the diagnostic "gold standard" for achalasia and should follow endoscopy and a timed barium esophagogram (TBE) to evaluate dysphagia and exclude organic pathology. TBE typically shows a dilated, aperistaltic esophagus with a "bird-beak" narrowing at the EGJ, indicating a functional obstruction due to LES

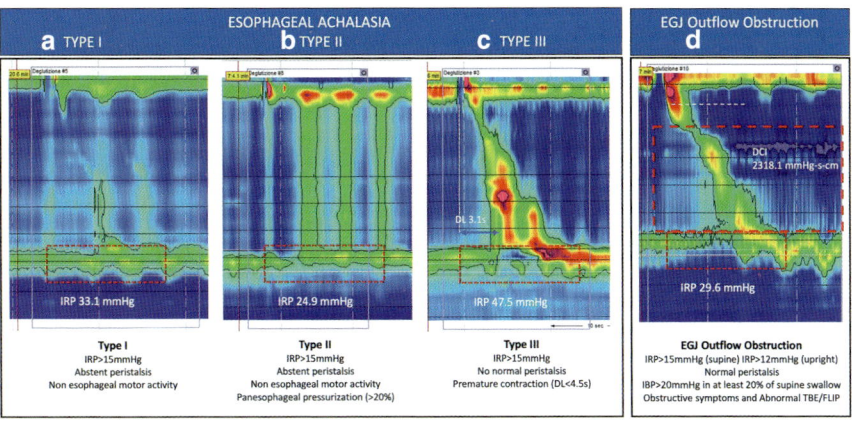

Fig. 4.2 Distinct pattern of achalasia: type I (**a**) is characterized by an integrated relaxation pressure (IRP) >15 mmHg, no peristalsis or esophageal contraction; type II (**b**) is characterized by IRP >15 mmHg and panesophageal pressurization (30 mmHg isobaric contour); type III (**c**) is characterized by IRP >15 mmHg, no normal peristalsis and at least 20% or more spastic contractions (distal latency <4.5 s); esophagogastric junction outflow obstruction (**d**) is characterized by IRP >15 mmHg (IRP >12 mmHg in upright position) and normal or weak peristalsis and increased intrabolus pressure (IBP) in 20% of supine swallows. *DL* distal latency, *EGJ* esophagogastric junction, *FLIP* functional lumen imaging probe, *TBE* timed barium esophagogram

non-relaxation. Upper endoscopy is performed to rule out malignancies near the EGJ, which may mimic achalasia. If no abnormalities or dilation are detected endoscopically, esophageal biopsies should be taken to exclude eosinophilic esophagitis.

HRM categorizes achalasia into three subtypes, each with distinct therapeutic implications. The median IRP should exceed 15 mmHg for diagnosis [1] (Fig. 4.2):

- Type I: Absence of esophageal body smooth muscle contractility, often reflecting advanced achalasia with muscle tone loss and esophageal dilation. In some cases, the esophagus is too dilated for pressure events to be recorded.
- Type II: Panesophageal compartmentalization of intrabolus pressure in at least 20% of swallows, with the smooth muscle retaining tone and responding to isobaric pressure to aid esophageal clearance.
- Type III: Premature contractions in over 20% of swallows, with shortened distal latency. The timing of peristalsis is abnormal, leading to premature contractions in the distal esophagus that lacks coordinated peristalsis.

The classification of achalasia into these subtypes is critical for selecting the appropriate therapeutic approach.

4.2.2 Esophagogastric Outflow Obstruction

Definition: In the latest version of the Chicago Classification (4.0), the definition of esophagogastric junction outflow obstruction (EGJ-OO) has been revised and now it may be considered a real esophageal motor disorder compared to the Chicago Classification 3.0 version in which it appeared as a manometric abnormality. The EGJ elevated relaxation pressure (IRP >15 mmHg) combined with intact or weak peristalsis is no longer considered conclusive for an EGJ-OO diagnosis (Fig. 4.2d).

Clinical presentation and diagnostic criteria: Patients with EGJ-OO typically present with obstructive symptoms, including dysphagia and non-cardiac chest pain. Elevated relaxation pressure (IRP >15 mmHg) in the supine position should also be confirmed in the upright position (IRP >12 mmHg), along with at least 20% of swallows showing increased intrabolus pressure (IBP). A definitive clinical diagnosis of EGJ-OO requires both manometric evidence of EGJ-OO and the presence of relevant clinical symptoms, supported by at least one additional diagnostic test indicating obstruction, such as TBE or functional lumen imaging probe (FLIP).

Since the classification of EGJ-OO as a motility disorder, nearly 10–15% of patients undergoing HRM have been identified with an EGJ-OO motility pattern. While some cases may progress toward achalasia or represent an achalasia variant, over one-third are clinically insignificant and may be attributed to benign causes, including mechanical factors, opioid use, or measurement artifacts, as detailed in the technical review of EGJ-OO. To prevent unnecessary treatments and improve patient outcomes, it is essential to distinguish which patients with manometric findings of EGJ-OO truly have obstructive physiology causing symptoms that warrant intervention.

Etiology and treatment: The exact cause of EGJ-OO remains unknown, and consensus on effective treatment is lacking. Before confirming a diagnosis of EGJ-OO, upper endoscopy with biopsies should be conducted to rule out eosinophilic esophagitis. Primary EGJ-OO may be managed with calcium channel blockers or nitrates. Some studies have reported positive outcomes following pneumatic dilation, similar to the approach used for achalasia. Recently, an Italian study from the Padua Esophageal Surgical Team presented the first series of patients with EGJ-OO successfully treated with Heller-Dor myotomy.

Moreover, the recent Padua Consensus Report (a multi-disciplinary international working group) developed consensus on the role of HRM pre- and post-antireflux surgery (ARS), and a postoperative classification to interpret HRM findings. This consensus stated that the LES obstruction, as defined by the updated manometric criteria of EGJ-OO in Chicago Classification version 4.0, must be addressed prior to undertaking ARS.

4.3 Disorders of Peristalsis

4.3.1 Aperistalsis

Definition: Aperistalsis, or absent peristalsis, is characterized by normal EGJ relaxation (IRP <15 mmHg) combined with failed esophageal contractions (100% with DCI <100 mmHg·s·cm) (Fig. 4.3a).

Aperistalsis often occurs as a secondary manifestation of systemic diseases, such as scleroderma—a connective tissue disorder frequently affecting the smooth

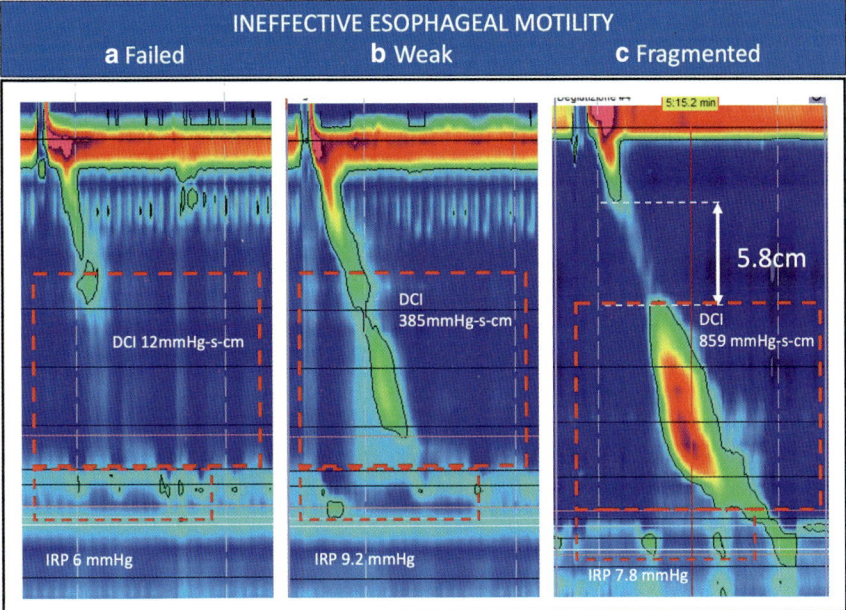

Fig. 4.3 Disorders of peristalsis with reduced contractile vigor or integrity of peristalsis. These include absent contractility or ineffective esophageal motility (either related to reduced contractile vigor or fragmented peristalsis). When the distal contractile integral (DCI) is <100 mmHg·s·cm (failed contraction; **a**) in 100% of wet swallows it is diagnostic for absent contractility. Ineffective esophageal motility (IEM) is characterized by ≥50% of failed peristalsis or >70% of weak peristalsis (**b**) with a normal integrated relaxation pressure (IRP). In the third example of IEM (**c**), the DCI is normal with a fragmentation in peristalsis of >5 cm in the setting of a normal IRP

muscle of the esophagus. Contrast radiography typically reveals a partially dilated, aperistaltic esophagus with some barium retention and retrograde bolus movement. Patients commonly present with symptoms like heartburn or regurgitation, which may lead to an initial diagnosis of GERD. Other systemic diseases, including systemic lupus erythematosus and polymyositis, can also affect esophageal motility by involving smooth muscle function.

A differential diagnosis between aperistalsis and type I achalasia is essential, as some cases of type I achalasia exhibit normal IRP values (<15 mmHg). This assessment should include a thorough clinical evaluation, endoscopy, and barium swallow study. Multiple diagnostic tests are recommended to confirm aperistalsis before making a final diagnosis.

4.3.2 Ineffective Esophageal Motility

Definition and diagnosis: Prior iterations of the Chicago Classification categorized ineffective esophageal motility (IEM) and fragmented peristalsis as minor motility disorders. In the latest version (4.0), fragmented peristalsis has been incorporated into the definition of IEM, and the diagnostic criteria for IEM have become more stringent in response to recent data. Consequently, the Chicago Classification version 4.0 no longer differentiates between major and minor motility disorders.

To confirm a diagnosis of IEM, there must be more than 70% ineffective swallows (either weak or failed) or at least 50% failed peristaltic contractions. An ineffective swallow includes either failed peristalsis (DCI <100 mmHg·s·cm; Fig. 4.3a), weak contractions (DCI ≥100 mmHg·s·cm but <450 mmHg·s·cm; Fig. 4.3b), or fragmented swallows (Fig. 4.3c). Fragmented peristalsis is characterized by normal DCI (>450 mmHg·s·cm) with large breaks (>5 cm) along a 20 mmHg isobaric contour [1, 4].

Epidemiology: IEM is the most frequently observed motility abnormality in routine esophageal manometry, with a prevalence estimated between 20% and 30%. Among patients presenting with esophageal dysphagia, IEM prevalence is reported to be as high as 51%. In GERD, IEM is present in approximately 50% of cases and is associated with increased acid exposure time on 24-hour pH monitoring, especially in the recumbent position, likely due to impaired esophageal clearance.

IEM is also commonly linked to conditions such as Barrett's esophagus, diabetic neuropathy, acute alcohol abuse, eosinophilic esophagitis, and autoimmune diseases affecting the esophagus (e.g., scleroderma) [4]. Currently, there is no effective treatment to enhance esophageal motility. Although buspirone and itiopride have shown potential in recent clinical trials, they are not yet available in Italy. Large-scale clinical trials are necessary to further elucidate the pathophysiology and clinical impact of these minor esophageal peristaltic disorders on patient symptoms.

4.3.3 Distal Esophageal Spasm

Definition: Distal esophageal spasm (DES) is identified using HRM when the IRP is below 15 mmHg, and 20% or more of swallows exhibit premature contractions, indicated by a DL of less than 4.5 seconds during 10 wet swallows (Fig. 4.4a).

Epidemiology: DES is a rare esophageal motility disorder. Studies from specialized centers indicate a prevalence of approximately 3–9% in large adult patient populations undergoing esophageal motility evaluations. The average age at diagnosis is around 60 years, with a slightly higher incidence in females (55%).

Etiology: The underlying cause of DES remains unclear, and the clinical presentation typically includes dysphagia and chest pain. In some cases, DES presents with a characteristic "corkscrew" appearance on barium radiography.

Histopathological data on DES are limited, as patients with this disorder rarely undergo autopsy. Some research suggests that DES is associated with impaired neural inhibition. Experimental studies in both animals and humans indicate that inhibition of nitric oxide (NO) activity can induce simultaneous contractions in the distal esophagus, a pattern characteristic of DES, while administration of NO appears to reverse this effect. DES has also been occasionally observed in patients with gastroesophageal symptoms.

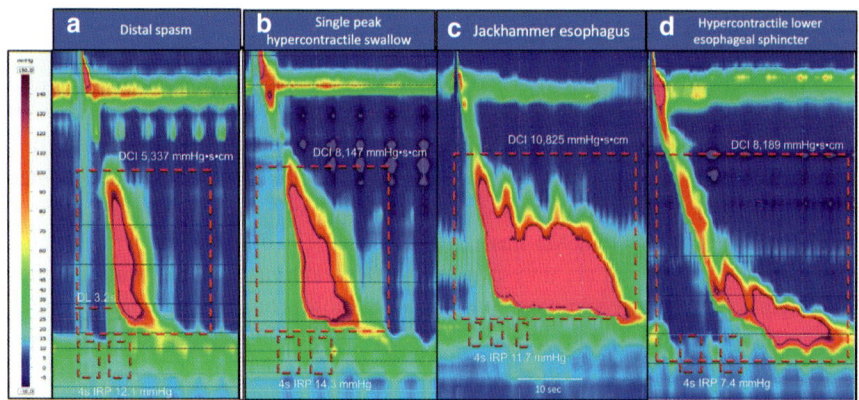

Fig. 4.4 Disorders of peristalsis with esophageal spasticity or hypercontractility. These include distal esophageal spasm or hypercontractile esophagus. In this example of distal esophageal spasm (**a**), the distal contractile integral (DCI) is normal with a reduced distal latency (DL <4.5 s) and normal integrated relaxation pressure (IRP). Hypercontractile esophagus includes sub-groups: single peak hypercontractile swallow (**b**), hypercontractile with jackhammer esophagus (**c**) characterized by chaotic propagation of the wave and repetitive contraction, and hypercontractile with lower esophageal sphincter (LES) after contraction (**d**)

4.3.4 Hypercontractile Esophagus

Definition and diagnosis: Hypercontractile esophagus is a unique manometric condition characterized by abnormally vigorous peristaltic contractions, sometimes accompanied by exaggerated LES after-contractions, in the absence of mechanical obstruction. A definitive manometric diagnosis requires that at least 20% of supine swallows exhibit hypercontractility, with a DCI exceeding 8000 mmHg·s·cm (Fig. 4.4b–d).

Hypercontractile esophagus can be categorized into three main subtypes: (1) single-peaked hypercontractile swallows (Fig. 4.4b), (2) "jackhammer" swallows characterized by repeated and prolonged contractions, particularly in the post-peak phase (Fig. 4.4c), and (3) hypercontractile swallows with strong LES after-contractions (Fig. 4.4d). These contractions, often located in the distal two-thirds of the esophageal body and sometimes the LES, may or may not synchronize with respiration [1, 5].

Pathophysiology: Currently, there is scanty histopathological information available to aid in the characterization of this motor abnormality. The pathophysiology is complex and not fully understood, although it is thought that hypercontractility may result from an imbalance between excitatory and inhibitory neural input. Additionally, spontaneous contractions may occur, possibly triggered by acetylcholine discharge independently of swallowing.

Hypercontractile esophagus is often observed in conjunction with other conditions, including EGJ-OO, GERD, or eosinophilic esophagitis. The primary symptom reported is chest pain, which requires evaluation to rule out cardiac origins.

Dysphagia is also present in approximately 30–60% of cases, though weight loss is uncommon.

Management: Currently, there is no consensus on optimal management strategies for hypercontractile esophagus or related conditions such as DES. First-line treatments in clinical practice include slow-releasing nitrates and endoscopic injection of botulinum toxin. Low-dose antidepressants may be considered for selected patients, with dosage adjustments over time to achieve symptom relief. Peroral endoscopic myotomy (POEM) has been proposed for cases of hypercontractile esophageal disorders that are unresponsive to medical treatment, particularly when dysphagia is the primary symptom; early reports show promising outcomes, though long-term efficacy data are lacking.

References

1. Yadlapati R, Kahrilas PJ, Fox MR, et al. Esophageal motility disorders on high-resolution manometry: Chicago classification version 4.0©. Neurogastroenterol Motil. 2021;33(1):e14058.
2. Gyawali CP, Roman S, Bredenoord AJ, et al. Classification of esophageal motor findings in gastro-esophageal reflux disease: conclusions from an international consensus group. Neurogastroenterol Motil. 2017;29(12):e13104.
3. Yadlapati R, Pandolfino JE, Fox MR, et al. What is new in Chicago classification version 4.0? Neurogastroenterol Motil. 2021;33(1):e14053.
4. Gyawali CP, Zerbib F, Bhatia S, et al. Chicago classification update (V4.0): technical review on diagnostic criteria for ineffective esophageal motility and absent contractility. Neurogastroenterol Motil. 2021;33(8):e14134.
5. Chen JW, Savarino E, Smout A, et al. Chicago classification update (v4.0): technical review on diagnostic criteria for hypercontractile esophagus. Neurogastroenterol Motil. 2021;33(6):e14115.

Open Access This chapter is licensed under the terms of the Creative Commons Attribution-NonCommercial 4.0 International License (http://creativecommons.org/licenses/by-nc/4.0/), which permits any noncommercial use, sharing, adaptation, distribution and reproduction in any medium or format, as long as you give appropriate credit to the original author(s) and the source, provide a link to the Creative Commons license and indicate if changes were made.

The images or other third party material in this chapter are included in the chapter's Creative Commons license, unless indicated otherwise in a credit line to the material. If material is not included in the chapter's Creative Commons license and your intended use is not permitted by statutory regulation or exceeds the permitted use, you will need to obtain permission directly from the copyright holder.

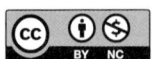

Esophageal pH and pH-Impedance Monitoring

5

Edoardo Vincenzo Savarino and Luisa Bertin

5.1 Indications and Contraindications

Reflux monitoring, including esophageal pH impedance testing, is crucial for evaluating various clinical scenarios. Ideally, pH monitoring should be conducted off proton pump inhibitors (PPIs) or potassium-competitive acid blockers to accurately demonstrate abnormal reflux, particularly when assessing atypical symptoms such as cough or, together with high-resolution manometry, prior to surgical or endoscopic interventions such as surgical or endoscopic fundoplication, non-ablative radiofrequency treatment, transoral incisionless fundoplication, antireflux mucosectomy, and anti-reflux mucosal ablation [1–3]. Reflux monitoring is also valuable for distinguishing functional gastrointestinal disorders, such as reflux hypersensitivity (RH) and functional heartburn (FH), which can mimic gastroesophageal reflux disease (GERD) and to exclude GERD in patients with symptoms compatible with globus or functional dysphagia [4]. Furthermore, emerging evidence indicates that reflux monitoring might be advantageous for individuals undergoing bariatric surgery, aiding in the selection of the optimal surgical approach [5–7].

Wireless pH testing should be the first choice in these cases, particularly for patients who cannot tolerate catheter-based pH studies [1]. For those with persistent symptoms not fully responsive to PPI therapy, pH impedance studies performed on optimized anti-secretory therapy can help differentiate between refractory GERD and disturbances related to gut-brain interactions [1, 4]. This distinction is important when considering potentially irreversible anti-reflux interventions. Additionally, pH impedance monitoring is useful for evaluating suspected rumination syndrome or frequent belching [1, 4]. It helps differentiate rumination syndrome from GERD-related regurgitation and distinguishes supragastric belching from gastric belching in order to tailor cognitive behavior therapy. Contraindications for reflux monitoring include significant anatomical abnormalities (e.g., esophageal strictures or large varices), severe coagulopathy, recent esophageal or upper gastrointestinal surgery, and patients' intolerance. Relative contraindications include recent esophageal bleeding, active throat infections, and conditions affecting patient compliance. For wireless pH monitoring, considerations include pregnancy, known gastrointestinal tract stenosis, and the need for an MRI scan within 30 days.

5.2 Methodology of pHmetry and pH-Impedance Monitoring

5.2.1 Equipment

The equipment of ambulatory esophageal reflux monitoring consists of a monitoring catheter or capsule, a portable recorder, and a data processing system.

5.2.1.1 Catheters

A pH monitoring catheter is equipped with a pH sensor, which includes a reference electrode at a constant potential and an indicator electrode sensitive to hydrogen ion concentration. The number of sensors or electrodes in a probe is referred to as "channels", with single-channel, dual-channel, and multichannel probes available to meet clinical or research needs. Changes in potential difference between the electrodes indicate pH value alterations, with data stored in a portable recorder and processed into real-time pH variation curves.

A multichannel intraluminal impedance and pH monitoring (MII-pH) catheter consists of one or two pH electrodes placed in the distal esophagus and at least eight metal rings forming impedance-measuring channels spaced along the esophagus [8]. MII-pH monitoring detects the physical and chemical characteristics of reflux episodes, including acidic, weakly acidic, and weakly alkaline reflux. It also provides detailed reflux profiles, including extent, velocity, clearance time, and bolus direction. The extent of reflux is classified based on how far it travels up the esophagus, with proximal reflux reaching 15 cm above the lower esophageal sphincter (LES).

Accurate placement of the pH catheter is crucial for reliable esophageal reflux monitoring. The procedure begins by assessing both nostrils to select the one with the clearer passage. After applying a local anesthetic, the catheter is gently inserted through the chosen nostril and guided towards the posterior pharynx. To facilitate the catheter's passage, the patient may be instructed to lower their head and, if needed, swallow to help move the probe through the oropharynx. The pH sensor should ideally be positioned 5 cm above the upper border of the LES. This placement, established during the development of the test, ensures that the sensor does not slip into the proximal stomach during esophageal contractions with swallowing or fail to detect reflux episodes if positioned too high in the esophagus [9, 10]. While manometry is commonly used to guide catheter placement, alternative methods such as radiography, endoscopy, or the pH "step-up" technique can be utilized if manometry is not available [11].

Once the catheter is in place, it is secured with a tape. The recorder, which should be worn around the waist or over the shoulder, is then used to track the patient's symptoms, meals, body position, and medication use. To ensure the accuracy and consistency of the data, a minimum of 16 hours of catheter-based monitoring is required [12–15]. Once the recording is finished and the catheter is removed, the data is transferred to a computer for subsequent analysis.

5.2.1.2 Wireless pH Monitoring

The core component is a small, biocompatible capsule containing a pH electrode, battery, and transmitter. The capsule attaches to the esophageal mucosa and transmits pH data to an external receiver, a portable recorder [16]. Two commercially available systems, Bravo™ and alpHaONE, offer different dimensions, weights, working durations, and sampling frequencies.

The capsule is usually placed transorally under endoscopic guidance for optimal comfort and accuracy. However, if necessary, it can also be positioned transnasally after identifying the LES using manometry. The capsule should be positioned approximately 6 cm above the Z-line or 9 cm above the LES, adjusted for the route taken [16, 17]. Figure 5.1 illustrates the variations in placement among the available devices.

Once the desired location is confirmed, the capsule is positioned using a delivery device. The capsule is attached to the esophageal wall by applying suction to draw tissue into the capsule's chamber. After placement, the delivery device is carefully removed.

Patients are generally provided with either a paper diary or an electronic device to log activities such as mealtime, position changes and their symptoms, with each

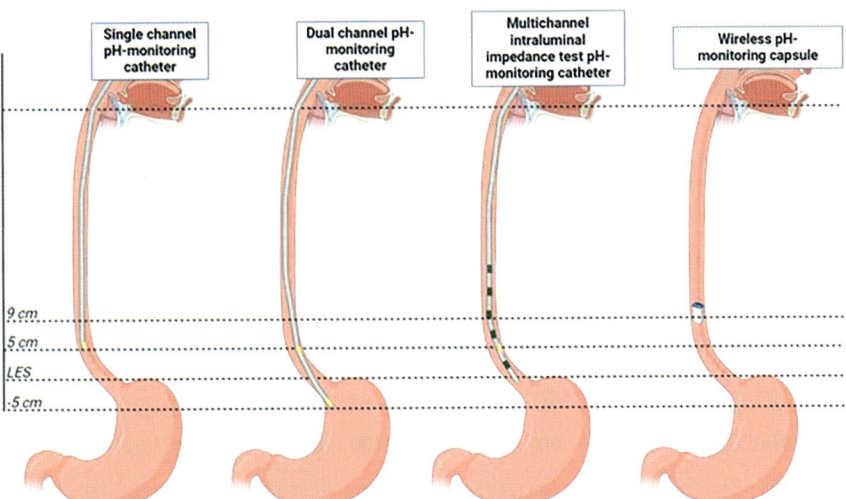

Fig. 5.1 Placement of catheter-based and wireless esophageal reflux monitoring equipment. The figure depicts the positioning of various reflux monitoring devices relative to the lower esophageal sphincter (LES). Yellow highlights indicate the location of the pH electrode, while green denotes the impedance electrode. (Created with Biorender.com [Last accessed 15/07/2024])

symptom noted along with its precise time of occurrence. The capsule will detach naturally, and it is disposable. X-ray confirmation of capsule passage may be considered in specific situations, such as patient concern or prolonged retention.

5.2.2 Analysis and Interpretation of pH Measurement and Impedance Analysis

5.2.2.1 Pre-analysis and Visual Inspection

Before analyzing pH- and pH-impedance recordings, it is important to conduct a visual inspection to rule out technical issues that might affect accuracy, such as recording gaps during mealtimes or prolonged periods of low pH values, gradual changes in pH values that may indicate failed calibration or damaged sensors, or misplacement of the pH electrode affecting measurements.

Automated analysis might overestimate non-acid reflux or inaccurately calculate reflux-symptom associations, necessitating manual review [18, 19]. Therefore, it is recommended to perform manual validation afterwards using a 5-minute or 2-minute time window to confirm or exclude reflux episodes and swallowing events and manual editing of data before final analysis. Challenges include the tedious nature of visual data inspection and limitations of current software, particularly in cases of severe esophagitis or Barrett's esophagus causing very low baseline levels [20].

A recent update to the original GERD Consensus diagnostic criteria has been published in the Lyon Consensus 2.0, which outlines criteria for both diagnosing and excluding GERD [1]. The main parameters assessed through pH-monitoring and pH-impedance monitoring are detailed below and summarized in Table 5.1, together with their commonly accepted cutoffs.

5.2.2.2 Acid Exposure Time

Acid exposure time (AET) is a key metric for diagnosing acid reflux, with a cutoff of pH <4.0 being widely accepted when using both catheter-based and catheter-free devices. This threshold is chosen because pepsin's proteolytic activity decreases in solutions with a pH above 4.0, and reflux symptoms commonly occur when intraesophageal pH drops below 4.0 [21, 24, 25]. AET is accurately calculated automatically through analysis software [26].

5.2.2.3 Number of Reflux Episodes

The total number of reflux episodes includes all types of reflux events [1, 4, 27]. Accurate interpretation of pH-impedance data often necessitates manual verification, as automated systems may overestimate the number of episodes. According to the Lyon Consensus 2.0, fewer than 40 reflux episodes per day suggest a lower likelihood of pathological GERD, while more than 80 episodes per day may indicate objective GERD [1]. However, these thresholds are not definitive for predicting therapy response or determining the need for surgery. In patients with confirmed GERD, a combination of an AET greater than 4% and more than 80 reflux episodes per day may signify refractory GERD [1].

Table 5.1 Main parameters evaluated with pH-monitoring and pH-impedance monitoring

	Catheter-based pHmetry	Impedance-pH monitoring	Wireless pHmetry
Duration of the procedure (hours)	24	24	48–96
AET (%) [1]	AET >6.0	AET >6.0 in patients with unproven GERD; AET >4% (combined with >80 reflux episodes/day) in patients with proven GERD [1]	AET >6.0% for ≥2 days
Total reflux episodes (acidic, weakly acidic, and weakly alkaline reflux) (n)	N/A	>80 in patients with unproven GERD; >80 (combined with AET >4%) in patients with proven GERD [1]	N/A
Symptom index (%) [1]	≥50	≥50	≥50
Symptom association probability (%) [1]	≥95	≥95	≥95
DeMeester score [21, 22]	≥14.72	≥14.72	≥14.72
Post-reflux swallow-induced peristaltic wave index (%) [23]	N/A	>61	N/A
Mean nocturnal baseline impedance (Ω)	N/A	<1500	N/A

AET acid exposure time, *GERD* gastroesophageal reflux disease

5.2.2.4 Symptom Association

To link symptoms with reflux episodes, clinical practice commonly employs tools such as the Symptom index (SI) and Symptom association probability (SAP) [28–30]. The SI measures the percentage of symptoms that occur within 5 minutes of a reflux event, divided by the total number of symptoms [21]. However, the SI does not account for the total number of reflux episodes, meaning a patient with numerous reflux episodes but only one symptomatic event could still have an SI of 100%. In contrast, the SAP uses statistical analysis to determine whether the association between reflux events and symptoms is likely due to chance. A SAP value greater than 95% indicates a less than 5% probability that the observed association is random, and is thus considered positive. The Lyon Consensus 2.0 on ambulatory reflux monitoring highlights that combining SI and SAP provides the most clinically relevant insights. These metrics are particularly important for distinguishing between reflux hypersensitivity and functional heartburn in patients with normal AET, where the former is characterized by a positive symptom-reflux association and the latter by a negative association [1, 4].

5.2.2.5 DeMeester Score

The DeMeester score is a comprehensive metric for assessing acid exposure that combines total AET, upright and supine AET, reflux episodes, and the longest acidic reflux episode. Most commercial pH monitoring software automatically calculates and reports this score, along with individual exposure times. While the DeMeester score helps address some of the variability related to sex and age seen with simple

AET, scores exceeding 14.72 generally indicate pathological acid exposure but do not account for symptom-reflux associations [21, 22]. Notably, this score has not been included in the original Lyon Consensus or the Lyon Consensus 2.0 guidelines for GERD diagnosis [1, 31].

5.2.2.6 Post-reflux Swallow-Induced Peristaltic Wave and Its Index

Esophageal clearance occurs in two distinct phases. The first phase is characterized by a secondary peristaltic wave, which is initiated by stretch receptors to clear volume from the esophagus. The second phase involves a primary peristaltic wave, triggered by an esophago-salivary vagal reflex, which delivers salivary bicarbonate and epidermal growth factor to the distal esophageal mucosa, thereby providing chemical clearance and restoring a neutral pH [32]. The post-reflux swallow-induced peristaltic waves (PSPWs) reflect this second phase of chemical clearance. In MII-pH monitoring, PSPWs are identified by an antegrade 50% drop in impedance from the pre-swallow baseline, starting at the most proximal impedance site and reaching all distal sites, followed by at least a 50% return to baseline at all distal sites [32, 33]. The PSPW index (PSPWI), calculated as the number of PSPWs divided by the total number of reflux episodes, is manually computed, with a value below 61% considered abnormal and indicative of potential pathological reflux [23]. While the Lyon Consensus 2.0 guidelines do not incorporate PSPW analysis in the diagnosis of GERD, it is recognized as a valuable research tool. PSPW analysis can be particularly useful for phenotyping GERD, as it has been found to be elevated in PPI-refractory GERD patients with esophagitis [1].

5.2.2.7 Mean Nocturnal Baseline Impedance

Exposure of the esophageal mucosa to harmful agents and the resulting mucosal damage may lead to a decrease in transepithelial electrical resistance [34]. Mean nocturnal baseline impedance (MNBI), measured during sleep, reflects esophageal mucosal integrity. There are two methods for calculating baseline impedance: it can be derived from the average of three 10-minute intervals between 1:00 and 3:00 a.m., or from the average of the entire nocturnal recumbent period [35, 36]. The calculation currently needs to be done manually [37, 38]. An MNBI of less than 1500 Ω suggests impaired mucosal integrity and supports the diagnosis of GERD, whereas an MNBI greater than 2500 Ω suggests normal mucosa and argues against pathological GERD, as was recently stated by the Lyon Consensus 2.0, and is particularly valuable when AET results are inconclusive [1].

References

1. Gyawali CP, Yadlapati R, Fass R, et al. Updates to the modern diagnosis of GERD: Lyon consensus 2.0. Gut. 2024;73:361–71.
2. Roman S, Gyawali CP, Savarino E, et al. Ambulatory reflux monitoring for diagnosis of gastroesophageal reflux disease: update of the Porto consensus and recommendations from an international consensus group. Neurogastroenterol Motil. 2017;29:1–15.
3. Lopes SO, Gonçalves AR, Macedo G, Santos-Antunes J. Endoscopic treatment of gastroesophageal reflux: a narrative review. Porto Biomed J. 2023;8:e226.

4. Aziz Q, Fass R, Gyawali CP, et al. Esophageal disorders. Gastroenterology. 2016;150:1368–79.
5. DuPree CE, Blair K, Steele SR, Martin MJ. Laparoscopic sleeve gastrectomy in patients with preexisting gastroesophageal reflux disease: a national analysis. JAMA Surg. 2014;149:328–34.
6. Abdulkhaleq MM, Alshugaig RS, Farhan DA, et al. Prevalence and associated factors of gastroesophageal reflux disease after laparoscopic sleeve gastrectomy. Cureus. 2024;16:e57921.
7. Trujillo AB, Sagar D, Amaravadhi AR, et al. Incidence of post-operative gastro-esophageal reflux disorder in patients undergoing laparoscopic sleeve gastrectomy: a systematic review and meta-analysis. Obes Surg. 2024;34:1874–84.
8. Sifrim D. Acid, weakly acidic and non-acid gastro-oesophageal reflux: differences, prevalence and clinical relevance. Eur J Gastroenterol Hepatol. 2004;16:823–30.
9. Johnson LF, Demeester TR. Twenty-four-hour pH monitoring of the distal esophagus. A quantitative measure of gastroesophageal reflux. Am J Gastroenterol. 1974;62:325–32.
10. Anggiansah A, Sumboonnanonda K, Wang J, et al. Significantly reduced acid detection at 10 centimeters compared to 5 centimeters above lower esophageal sphincter in patients with acid reflux. Am J Gastroenterol. 1993;88:842–6.
11. Klauser AG, Schindlbeck NE, Müller-Lissner SA. Esophageal 24-h pH monitoring: is prior manometry necessary for correct positioning of the electrode? Am J Gastroenterol. 1990;85:1463–7.
12. Pandolfino JE, Vela MF. Esophageal-reflux monitoring. Gastrointest Endosc. 2009;69(917–30):930.e1.
13. Trudgill NJ, Sifrim D, Sweis R, et al. British Society of Gastroenterology guidelines for oesophageal manometry and oesophageal reflux monitoring. Gut. 2019;68:1731–50.
14. Xiao Y, Wu JCY, Lu C-L, et al. Clinical practice guidelines for esophageal ambulatory reflux monitoring in Chinese adults. J Gastroenterol Hepatol. 2022;37:812–22.
15. Savarino E, Frazzoni M, Marabotto E, et al. A SIGE-SINGEM-AIGO technical review on the clinical use of esophageal reflux monitoring. Dig Liver Dis. 2020;52(9):966–80.
16. Pandolfino JE, Schreiner MA, Lee TJ, et al. Comparison of the Bravo wireless and Digitrapper catheter-based pH monitoring systems for measuring esophageal acid exposure. Am J Gastroenterol. 2005;100:1466–76.
17. Lacy BE, O'Shana T, Hynes M, et al. Safety and tolerability of transoral Bravo capsule placement after transnasal manometry using a validated conversion factor. Am J Gastroenterol. 2007;102:24–32.
18. Roman S, des Varannes SB, Pouderoux P, et al. Ambulatory 24-h oesophageal impedance-pH recordings: reliability of automatic analysis for gastro-oesophageal reflux assessment. Neurogastroenterol Motil. 2006;18:978–86.
19. Zentilin P, Dulbecco P, Savarino E, et al. Combined multichannel intraluminal impedance and pH-metry: a novel technique to improve detection of gastro-oesophageal reflux literature review. Dig Liver Dis. 2004;36:565–9.
20. Johnsson F, Joelsson B. Reproducibility of ambulatory oesophageal pH monitoring. Gut. 1988;29:886–9.
21. Pohl D, Tutuian R. Reflux monitoring: pH-metry, Bilitec and oesophageal impedance measurements. Best Pract Res Clin Gastroenterol. 2009;23:299–311.
22. Johnsson F, Joelsson B, Isberg PE. Ambulatory 24 hour intraesophageal pH-monitoring in the diagnosis of gastroesophageal reflux disease. Gut. 1987;28:1145–50.
23. Frazzoni L, Frazzoni M, de Bortoli N, et al. Postreflux swallow-induced peristaltic wave index and nocturnal baseline impedance can link PPI-responsive heartburn to reflux better than acid exposure time. Neurogastroenterol Motil. 2017;29(11):e13116.
24. Piper DW, Fenton BH. pH stability and activity curves of pepsin with special reference to their clinical importance. Gut. 1965;6:506–8.
25. Spencer J. Prolonged pH recording in the study of gastro-oesophageal reflux. Br J Surg. 1969;56:912–4.
26. Bredenoord AJ, Weusten BLAM, Timmer R, Smout AJPM. Reproducibility of multichannel intraluminal electrical impedance monitoring of gastroesophageal reflux. Am J Gastroenterol. 2005;100:265–9.

27. Hong S-KS, Vaezi MF. Gastroesophageal reflux monitoring: pH (catheter and capsule) and impedance. Gastrointest Endosc Clin N Am. 2009;19:1–22.
28. Wiener GJ, Richter JE, Copper JB, et al. The symptom index: a clinically important parameter of ambulatory 24-hour esophageal pH monitoring. Am J Gastroenterol. 1988;83:358–61.
29. Breumelhof R, Smout AJ. The symptom sensitivity index: a valuable additional parameter in 24-hour esophageal pH recording. Am J Gastroenterol. 1991;86:160–4.
30. Weusten BL, Roelofs JM, Akkermans LM, et al. The symptom-association probability: an improved method for symptom analysis of 24-hour esophageal pH data. Gastroenterology. 1994;107:1741–5.
31. Gyawali CP, Kahrilas PJ, Savarino E, et al. Modern diagnosis of GERD: the Lyon Consensus. Gut. 2018;67:1351–62.
32. Frazzoni M, Manta R, Mirante VG, et al. Esophageal chemical clearance is impaired in gastro-esophageal reflux disease–a 24-h impedance-pH monitoring assessment. Neurogastroenterol Motil. 2013;25(399–406):e295.
33. Vaezi MF, Choksi Y. Mucosal impedance: a new way to diagnose reflux disease and how it could change your practice. Am J Gastroenterol. 2017;112:4–7.
34. Woodland P, Al-Zinaty M, Yazaki E, Sifrim D. In vivo evaluation of acid-induced changes in oesophageal mucosa integrity and sensitivity in non-erosive reflux disease. Gut. 2013;62:1256–61.
35. Martinucci I, de Bortoli N, Savarino E, et al. Esophageal baseline impedance levels in patients with pathophysiological characteristics of functional heartburn. Neurogastroenterol Motil. 2014;26:546–55.
36. Hoshikawa Y, Sawada A, Sonmez S, et al. Measurement of esophageal nocturnal baseline impedance: a simplified method. J Neurogastroenterol Motil. 2020;26:241–7.
37. Savarino E, Marabotto E, Bodini G, et al. Advancements in the use of manometry and impedance testing for esophageal functional disorders. Expert Rev Gastroenterol Hepatol. 2019;13:425–35.
38. Frazzoni M, de Bortoli N, Frazzoni L, et al. The added diagnostic value of postreflux swallow-induced peristaltic wave index and nocturnal baseline impedance in refractory reflux disease studied with on-therapy impedance-pH monitoring. Neurogastroenterol Motil. 2017;29(3):e13116.

Open Access This chapter is licensed under the terms of the Creative Commons Attribution-NonCommercial 4.0 International License (http://creativecommons.org/licenses/by-nc/4.0/), which permits any noncommercial use, sharing, adaptation, distribution and reproduction in any medium or format, as long as you give appropriate credit to the original author(s) and the source, provide a link to the Creative Commons license and indicate if changes were made.

The images or other third party material in this chapter are included in the chapter's Creative Commons license, unless indicated otherwise in a credit line to the material. If material is not included in the chapter's Creative Commons license and your intended use is not permitted by statutory regulation or exceeds the permitted use, you will need to obtain permission directly from the copyright holder.

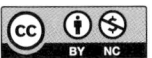

New Techniques of Endoscopy

Pier Alberto Testoni and Sabrina Testoni

6.1 Introduction

Gastroesophageal reflux disease (GERD) is a very common disorder that can be treated by medical, surgical, or endoluminal therapy. Proton pump inhibitors (PPIs) are the therapy of choice; however, several issues have been raised in the last years about PPI-based treatment of GERD and approximately up to 40% of patients with GERD are unsatisfied with PPI therapy [1–7]. For patients who have contraindications to long-term use of PPIs or medically refractory GERD, laparoscopic fundoplication or endoluminal interventions may be required. Surgical procedures for GERD create a flap valve by wrapping the gastric fundus around the gastroesophageal junction (so-called fundoplication). However, outcomes are suboptimal and there is a risk of long-lasting adverse events such as dysphagia, gas-bloat syndrome, and inability to vomit or belch [8]. In fact, considering all these drawbacks, patients suffering from a mild form of GERD are in general reluctant to undergo surgical repair of the valve. Concerns related to medical and surgical therapy of GERD have led to search for therapeutic endoluminal alternatives less invasive than surgery and free from drug-related side effects. Several techniques have been proposed in the past, but all were abandoned and are no longer available due to poor efficacy and safety issues. However, since the year 2001 novel endoluminal techniques have been introduced in clinical practice and proven effective in the treatment of GERD in selected patients, with an optimal safety profile.

P. A. Testoni (✉)
Vita Salute San Raffaele University, Milan, Italy
e-mail: pieralberto.testoni@gmail.com

S. Testoni
Gastroenterology Unit, IRCCS Policlinico San Donato, San Donato Milanese, Italy
e-mail: sabrina.testoni@grupposandonato.it

These techniques can be categorized into three categories:

1. Transoral incisionless fundoplication (TIF), aiming to reconstruct the lower esophageal sphincter (LES): EsophyX™ 2.0/Z (EndoGastric Solutions, Redmond, WA, USA), Medigus Ultrasonic Surgical Endostapler™ (MUSE™) (Medigus, Omer, Israel), and GERD-X™ (G-SURG GmbH, Seeon-Seebruck; Germany).
2. Mucosal resection/ablation for gastric cardia constriction: antireflux mucosectomy (ARMS) and antireflux mucosal ablation (ARMA).
3. Delivery of radiofrequency energy near the LES to increase its pressure (STRETTA®; Mederi Therapeutics, Norwalk, CT, USA).

6.2 Transoral Incisionless Fundoplication

TIF reconfigures the tissue to obtain a full-thickness gastroesophageal valve from inside the stomach, by means of serosa-to-serosa plications which include the muscle layers, mimicking a mean 180° up to 270° surgical fundoplication, depending on the technique adopted. The neo-valve is capable of boosting the barrier function of the LES with less discomfort and fewer side effects for the patient compared to surgery.

6.2.1 EsophyX™ 2.0/Z

EsophyX™ is the endoluminal platform with the greatest experience, with more than 25,000 TIF procedures performed so far worldwide, as reported by market data. This technique reduces the angle of His and a small hiatal hernia by constructing a 250°–300° (mean 270°) neo-valve. Four generations of EsophyX™ models have been produced over the years [9], but good clinical results have been obtained only with the 2.0 and Z models. The neo-valve is created by placing at least 20 polypropylene H-shaped fasteners transmurally across the esophagogastric tissue, 1 cm and 3 cm below the Z-line. Before deploying the fasteners, a torque is applied by rotation allowing part of the fundus to rotate around the esophageal wall and more tissue to be engaged by the stylet. Rolling the fundus over and around the distal esophagus increased by 30% the success rate of the procedure [10, 11]. The technique is able to reduce hiatal hernias ≤2.5 cm. Details of TIF by EsophyX Z™ are illustrated in Fig. 6.1. EsophyX™ 2.0/Z is currently the only endoluminal technique that fulfils four of the five principles reported for an effective antireflux surgery: it reduces hiatal hernia ≤2.5 cm; it elongates the intra-abdominal esophagus; it creates a fundoplication without strictures by approximating and tightening the fundus around the esophagus and recreating the dynamics of the angle of His; and it restores the gastroesophageal high-pressure zone.

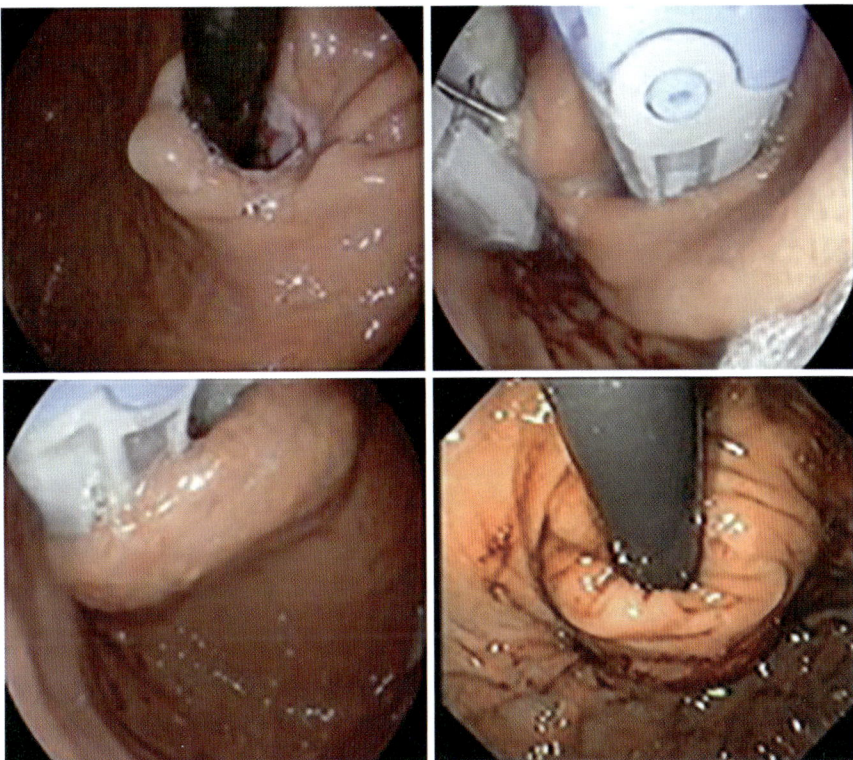

Fig. 6.1 Transoral fundoplication by EsophyX™ 2.0. With the gastroscope placed in a retroflexed position, tissue is drawn into the device with a helical tissue screw to create a valve. The fastener deployment process initiates on the far posterior and anterior sides of the esophagogastric valve adjacent to the lesser curvature and is then extended to the greater curvature, resulting in a new valve with a circumference of >240° and a length of 3 cm. Additional fasteners can be deployed to further reinforce the neo-valve. Before deploying fasteners a torque is applied by rotation allowing part of the fundus to rotate around the esophageal wall and more tissue to be engaged by the stylet

6.2.2 Medigus Ultrasonic Surgical Endostapler™ (MUSE™)

MUSE™ is no longer available in Europe and USA but currently used in China and Far East countries. It staples the fundus of the stomach to the esophagus below the diaphragm using three sets of five metal sutures, placed under an ultrasound-guided technique and a software program, mimicking a 3 cm-long, 180° anterior fundoplication [12, 13]. Details of the MUSE™ procedures are illustrated in Fig. 6.2. MUSE™ is unable to reduce hiatal hernia, differently from EsophyX™; hiatal hernia can be reduced only by applying a positive end-expiratory pressure (PEEP) of at least 5 mmHg (7.5 cm H_2O) with the patient intubated.

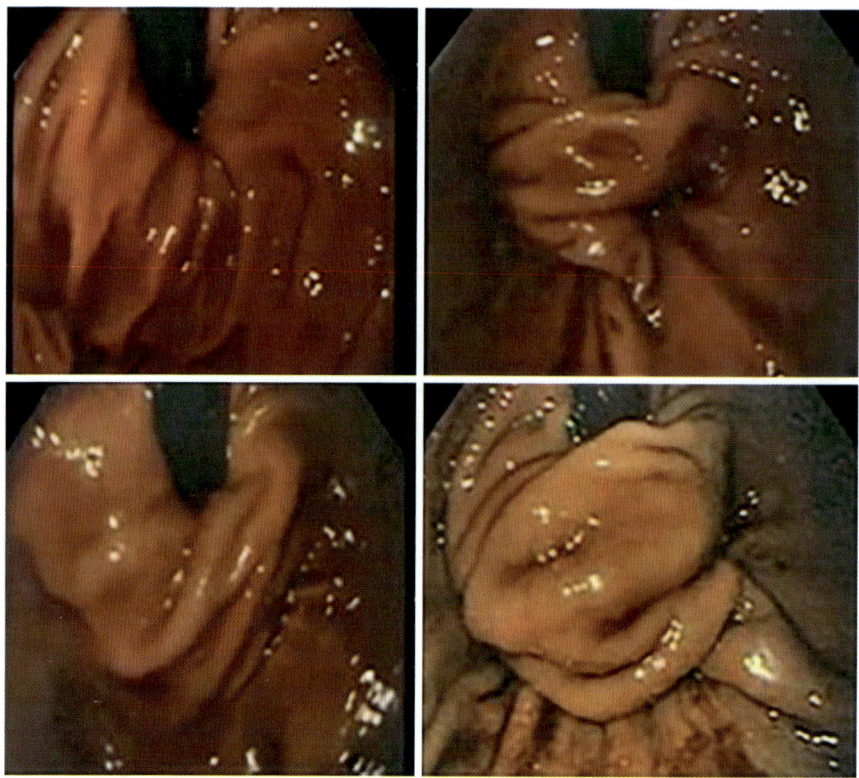

Fig. 6.2 Transoral fundoplication by MUSE™. The scope is retroflexed and pulled back to keep the cartridge approximately 3 cm above the gastroesophageal junction to clamp the tissue and place staples using the ultrasonic range finder. Stapling starts in the leftmost location; this is the anchoring point for the fundus and should be placed as far to the left of the esophagus as possible. The additional stapling locations should be within 60°–180°

6.2.3 GERD-X™

This is a modification of the original plicator device. The procedure is like that of EsophyX™ but creates an anterior fundoplication. Once the device is retroflexed into the gastric fundus, the plicator arms are opened and cardia tissue is gathered between the arms, with deployment of a pre-tied transmural pledgeted suture. The procedure can be repeated to deploy additional sutures for a tighter closure [14]. The device is presented in Fig. 6.3. The device is unable to reduce hiatal hernia.

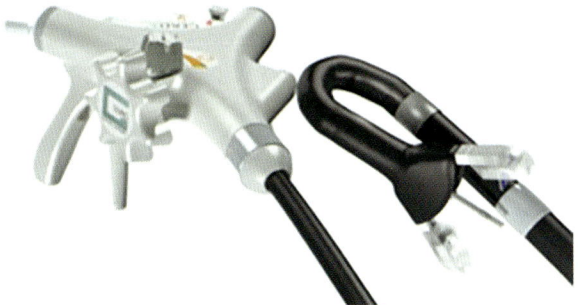

Fig. 6.3 Transoral fundoplicaton by GERD-X™. Once the device is retroflexed into the gastric fundus, the plicator arms are opened and the tissue retractor is advanced into the gastric cardia and pulled back to gather tissue between the arms of the plicator. The arms are then closed to deploy a pre-tied transmural pledgeted suture. The procedure can be repeated to deploy additional sutures for a tighter closure (G-SURG GmbH, GmbH, Seeon-Seebruck; Germany)

6.3 Antireflux Mucosectomy/Ablation

ARMS is a relatively novel endoscopic technique developed by Inoue et al. The idea came from the circumferential mucosal resection of Barrett's mucosa with high-grade dysplasia up to 2 cm of gastric cardia, resulting in reduced reflux symptoms. The procedure involves increasing the mucosal resection along the lesser curvature (1 cm in the esophagus and 2 cm in the stomach) using endoscopic mucosal resection techniques. The antireflux effect of ARMS is due to scar formation along the gastric side, resulting in a narrowed cardia opening. The first patients undergoing ARMS were treated by circumferential mucosal resection that allowed effective reduction of reflux episodes but was associated with a high incidence of strictures requiring dilation. A mucosal resection involving half to two-thirds of the circumference appeared to be a good compromise between effective treatment of reflux symptoms and risk of stricture. A pilot study of 10 patients showed a significant improvement of acid exposure time and DeMeester score, with all patients being able to discontinue PPI therapy [15].

ARMA was first used by Inoue et al. as additional treatment in a patient with post-ARMS insufficient shrinkage of the cardia opening resulting in unresolved symptoms. Ablation is carried out by argon beam using soft power, after creating a submucosal cushion to reduce the risk of perforation by thermal injury. It starts 0.5–1.0 cm above the Z-line and is extended up to 2.0 cm below in the stomach, along the lesser curvature. In general, ablation involves approximately 50% of mucosa, but its extension can be increased to two-thirds in cases with reduced LES basal pressure and severe esophagitis. Inoue et al. performed a pilot study of 12 patients: both the GERD health-related quality of life (GERD-HRQL) and DeMeester scores improved significantly [16]. Post-procedure dysphagia was reported only in one patient.

Both ARMS and ARMA cannot reduce hiatal hernia but have the advantage of being less costly than other endoscopic device-assisted antireflux procedures. However, long-term studies on larger series of patients are needed to validate this therapy.

6.4 Delivery of Radiofrequency (STRETTA®)

The STRETTA® system involves delivery of radiofrequency energy to muscles of the LES and gastric cardia using a catheter with a four-channel radiofrequency generator and a balloon-basket assembly with four nitinol needle electrodes at the tip. The energy is delivered to an area spanning 2 cm above and below the gastroesophageal junction. Radiofrequency energy is delivered at low frequency and power output with a temperature range of 65 °C–85 °C in the muscularis propria (Fig. 6.4). STRETTA® is assumed to work by causing collagen deposition with consequent submucosal fibrosis and hypertrophy of the LES muscle, which reduce wall distensibility of the gastroesophageal junction and the frequency and amplitude of post-prandial transient LES relaxations. STRETTA® also reduces esophageal sensitivity to refluxed acid, with a positive effect on pyrosis. Best candidates for STRETTA® treatment are patients suffering from GERD with predominant retrosternal pyrosis and hypersensitive esophagus [17]. The procedure should not be indicated in presence of hiatal hernia >2.0 cm, hypertonic motility disorders of the esophagus and severe esophagitis.

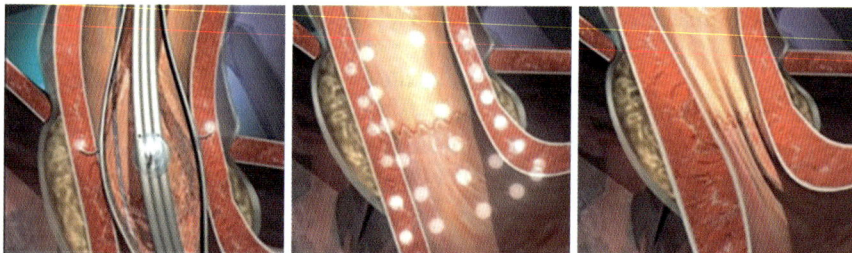

Fig. 6.4 Delivery of radiofrequency by STRETTA®. The balloon-basket assembly is advanced to the esophagogastric junction and then inflated to introduce the four needles into the muscularis propria layer. The energy is delivered to an area spanning 2 cm above and below the gastroesophageal junction. The procedure is repeated rotating the catheter by 45° to deliver energy to four additional sites, to treat the entire cardia circumference

6.5 Clinical Efficacy of Endoluminal Antireflux Therapies

To date, sufficient data to draw conclusions about the efficacy and safety of endoluminal antireflux procedures are available only for STRETTA® and EsophyX™ 2.0.

The efficacy of STRETTA® has been proven in two large meta-analyses of 1441 and 2468 patients, respectively, showing improvements in the GERD-HRQL score, reduction of acid exposure time, increased basal LES pressure, and safety [18, 19]. The long-term efficacy in terms of patient satisfaction and reduced PPI use has been reported over a 10-year follow-up [20]. However, a recent systematic meta-analysis including four randomized controlled trials and focusing on normalization of acid exposure time and ability to stop PPI as endpoints failed to find any significant difference between STRETTA® and sham therapy [21].

The efficacy and safety of TIF by EsophyX™ 2.0 have been documented in four meta-analyses [22–25] reporting significant improvement in symptomatic outcomes, patient satisfaction and PPI cessation. Functional findings, when reported, were assessed in three meta-analyses and showed that TIF with rotational technique was effective in reducing the mean esophageal acid exposure time, number of reflux episodes, and DeMeester score. One meta-analysis (9 studies, 868 patients) compared TIF with magnetic sphincter augmentation, reporting comparable outcomes [24]. Another meta-analysis including only long-term studies (>3 years), with TIF performed with both EsophyX™ 2.0 and MUSE™, showed that the symptomatic improvement achieved in the first three years was maintained over time up to ten years [25]. TIF with EsophyX™ 2.0/Z is a safe procedure. Severe adverse events (SAEs) have been reported in 2–2.5% of cases. More frequent SAEs were perforations, bleeding, pneumothorax and mediastinitis. Since 2008, the Manufacturer and User Facility Device Experience (MAUDE) FDA database reported a SAE rate of approximately 0.36%, with no mortalities, in over 25,000 TIF 2.0 procedures performed [26].

Data supporting the efficacy and safety of TIF performed by MUSE™ are limited. Long-term outcomes up to 3 and 5 years have been reported in four studies [12, 27–29]. A significant improvement of GERD-HRQL was reported in all the studies 6 months after the intervention and was maintained up to 5 years. PPI use was stopped in 69–84% of patients; satisfaction rate was reported in two studies and varied from 77% to 84%. The complication rate was similar to that reported for EsophyX™ 2.0, but the severity was higher, requiring surgical repair in several cases. Despite the good clinical results, few centers have adopted this technique because of the severity of SAEs. A recent study at our center comparing EsophyX™ 2.0 and MUSE™ reported similar technical success rates (98% and 97.8%, respectively) and moderate-severe adverse event rates (4.1% and 4.4%, respectively). However, the MUSE™-related adverse events were life-threatening. Outcomes in terms of GERD recurrence, PPI consumption and patient satisfaction were also similar [30]. Although TIF is nowadays proposed as an effective therapy in selected patients, the long-term outcomes need to be compared to those of laparoscopic Nissen and partial fundoplication, which still represent the gold standard treatment for refractory GERD, to draw definite conclusions about the real clinical efficacy of

Table 6.1 Long-term (5–10 years) clinical outcomes of transoral incisionless fundoplication (TIF), laparoscopic Nissen fundoplication (LNF) and laparoscopic partial fundoplication (LPF)

	TIF (9 studies; 308 patients)	LNF (8 studies; 497 patients)	LPF (8 studies; 442 patients)
GERD recurrence	22.6% (14.3%–32.3%)	22.7% (9.6%–37.8%)	20.5% (13.3%–29.7%)
Cessation of PPI therapy	69.8% (41.7%–84.6%)	59.3% (7.7%–91.9%)	70.1% (29.3%–96.7%)
Patients satisfied	76.8% (70.4%–86.7%)	81.3% (69.4%–89.4%)	75.5% (68.7%–91.8%)

GERD gastroesophageal reflux disease, *LNF* laparoscopic Nissen fundoplication, *LPF* laparoscopic partial fundoplication, *PPI* proton-pump inhibitor, *TIF* transoral incisionless fundoplication

TIF. To do this, we carried out a systematic literature review assessing GERD recurrence, cessation of PPI therapy and patient satisfaction, 5 to 10 years after the procedure, in patients who underwent TIF, laparoscopic Nissen and partial fundoplication. In fact, the outcomes proved to be substantially similar for the three fundoplication techniques, as reported in Table 6.1. A recent meta-analysis including 33 studies (4382 patients) and comparing the long-term outcomes of the different laparoscopic antireflux fundoplications, magnetic sphincter, STRETTA®, TIF, PPI and placebo in the treatment of GERD, showed a substantially similar efficacy on typical reflux symptoms and PPI use, and the lack of significant differences in the pre- and post-procedural LES basal pressure and pH variations [31].

Few data are available for the GERD-X™ procedure. Clinical efficacy has been assessed in three prospective studies including few patients, with a follow-up limited to only 3 and 12 months. All studies reported a significant improvement of the GERD-HRQL score and limited response in objective parameters (DeMeester score, esophageal acid exposure and LES basal pressure). The largest study (70 patients randomized to either GERD-X™ or a sham procedure) reported an improvement in total acid and non-acid reflux episodes in the GERD-X™ arm at 3 months but not at 12 months, compared to the sham procedure [32]. No major SAEs were noted in the three studies. The clinical efficacy of GERD-X™ needs to be confirmed in larger studies with longer follow-up periods; however, the impossibility to reduce hiatal hernia represents a limitation of this technique.

Outcomes of ARMS and ARMA are limited to 3 years and have been assessed in a recent meta-analysis including 15 nonrandomized studies (12 ARMS, n = 331; 3 ARMA, n = 130) [33]. ARMS and ARMA yielded similar clinical success rates, with significant improvements in GERD-HRQL score, recurrence of esophagitis, and acid exposure time. The pooled 6-month, 1- and 3-year mean clinical success rates were 78%, 72% and 73%, respectively, while the overall proportion of patients off PPIs at 1 year was 64%. The most common adverse event was dysphagia (11%), requiring dilation (7%). Four cases of perforation were recorded in patients undergoing ARMS. This poses the question of whether ARMA should replace ARMS, given that ablation achieved similar GERD control. However, the body of evidence is less for ARMA, and no head-to-head studies have been carried out. Again, studies on long-term outcomes are needed.

6.6 Which Patients Should Consider Endoluminal Therapy for GERD?

Patient selection for endoluminal therapy is critical. The patient must have a clear indication for an antireflux procedure, such as esophagitis or non-erosive esophagitis documented at functional investigation (NERD); hypersensitive esophagus is an indication as well, but the outcomes are more uncertain. Patients with functional heartburn should not be considered for invasive procedures. Patients should also respond at least partially to PPI therapy. Among patients with esophagitis, endoluminal techniques should be suggested in the presence of mild disease (grade A or B according to the Los Angeles classification), because no data are currently available on the efficacy of these procedures in more severe esophagitis, which has been considered an exclusion criterion in all protocol studies so far. As regards Barrett's esophagus endoluminal therapy may be suggested only in the presence of a short segment (≤ 3 cm), because data on long-segment disease are currently unavailable. To identify which patients are good candidates for the different antireflux treatments, several parameters should be considered: A) whether there is a hiatal hernia, what is its vertical and axial size, and whether it can reduce spontaneously or not. The axial and vertical length of the hiatal hernia can be assessed by an esophagogram or upper endoscopy; B) Hill's grade of the gastroesophageal junction. Hill's classification is the most effective way to quantify the crural opening and is best assessed during a retroflex view of the endoscope with active insufflation of 60 seconds at least; C) whether the LES needs to have a valve reconstruction; D) whether the right crus, which acts as a sling or noose around the gastroesophageal junction, needs to be tightened; E) whether there is impairment of esophageal motility (ineffective esophageal motility [IEM] according to the Chicago classification) and what is its severity. A Hill's grade 1 or 2 of the valve and a hiatal hernia up to 2.5 cm in length and 2.5 cm in axial diameter are acceptable for endoluminal therapy; more severe Hill's grades and sizes of hiatal hernia will most likely need a crural repair, which cannot be accomplished with endoluminal procedures alone. However, studies on TIF in presence of Hill's grades 3 and 4 are ongoing. In the presence of IEM, the Nissen fundoplication is in general not indicated to avoid post-interventional dysphagia, and partial laparoscopic fundoplication is preferred. In these patients TIF by EsophyX™ 2.0/Z creates a circumferential fundoplication (270°) like that obtained by the Nissen technique but without risks of dysphagia. However, the grade of IEM severity that would significantly affect post-TIF outcomes is still an unsettled issue. Among the available endoluminal therapies, current guidelines include only STRETTA® and TIF by EsophyX™ 2.0/Z, because for the other techniques evidence-based recommendations are lacking. Indications for endoluminal therapy are GERD persisting for at least 6 months, responsive or partially responsive to PPI therapy, with hiatal hernia ≤ 2.5 cm in length and Hill's grade 1–2 of the valve, in patients who are intolerant or have contraindication to PPI therapy, or require high dose maintenance therapy, or refuse it, as first choice instead of laparoscopic fundoplication.

6.7 Future Perspectives for Transoral Incisionless Fundoplication

With TIF by EsophyX™ 2.0/Z now established as an effective endoscopic antireflux procedure for selected patients with GERD, there are many clinical "settings" where TIF is being explored.

TIF has been performed along with concomitant laparoscopic hernia repair (cTIF), within a trend moving away from Nissen fundoplication due to high rates of postoperative gas-bloat syndrome and dysphagia. From a surgical technical point of view, performing laparoscopic repair of the hiatal defect alone avoids the more extensive dissection required to create the retroesophageal window where to reposition the bulk of the fundus, which may increase the risk of complications. The Food and Drug Administration (FDA) approved in 2017 cTIF in patients with hiatal hernia larger than 2 cm. Results of the first studies showed that after cTIF 74% to 90% of subjects were not using PPI and there were no adverse events related to laparoscopic surgery. Although this is an interesting trend, randomized clinical trials are required to establish cTIF efficacy and side effects compared with the standard Nissen or partial fundoplication.

TIF is being used after esophageal peroral endoscopic myotomy (E-POEM). Recent meta-analyses show that POEM achieves better improvement of dysphagia than Heller myotomy, with a 50% risk of developing GERD, which is similar for two procedures. The risk is reduced to 10% if a partial laparoscopic fundoplication is associated with Heller myotomy. In fact, a laparoscopic fundoplication is routinely performed along with Heller myotomy to prevent a GERD, which will occur in only about 50% of cases. A cost-effective strategy could be to reserve TIF only for those patients who develop post-POEM GERD. A strategy of pre-emptive TIF has been also suggested before E-POEM for type 1 achalasia patients with dilated and tortuous esophagus to "straighten" the esophagus by retracting more of the esophagus below the diaphragm in creation of the neo-valve.

TIF can be considered in obese patients before laparoscopic sleeve gastrectomy or endoscopic gastroplasty, given the higher rate of GERD with these procedures compared with Roux-en-Y gastric bypass (RYGB). Because TIF does not incorporate much of the gastric fundus, a gastrectomy or gastroplasty is still feasible after a TIF. This strategy may decrease the number of patients undergoing RYGB due to preoperative GERD. TIF post-gastrectomy is also possible, although it requires a sufficient gastric luminal diameter for the device to close.

Another potential field of application for TIF is Barrett's esophagus. To date only patients with short segment have undergone TIF but the numbers are too low to draw conclusions and no data are available for long-segment disease. In particular, TIF could be offered to patients with a previous history of Barrett's dysplasia who have reached complete remission of intestinal metaplasia by endoscopic resection and/or ablation but need lifelong use of PPIs.

References

1. Sharma N, Agrawal A, Freeman J, et al. An analysis of persistent symptoms in acid-suppressed patients undergoing impedance-pH monitoring. Clin Gastroenterol Hepatol. 2008;6:521–4.
2. Hershcovici T, Fass R. An algorithm for diagnosis and treatment of refractory ERD. Best Pract Res Clin Gastroenterol. 2010;24:923–36.
3. Cicala M, Emerenziani S, Guarino MPL, Ribolsi M. Proton pump inhibitor resistance, the real challenge in gastro-esophageal reflux disease. World J Gastroenterol. 2013;19:6529–35.
4. Rettura F, Bronzini F, Campigotto M, et al. Refractory gastroesophageal reflux disease: a management update. Front Med. 2021;8:1–19.
5. Grant AM, Cotton SC, Boachie C, et al. Minimal access surgery compared with medical management for gastro-oesophageal reflux disease: five-year follow-up of a randomised controlled trial (REFLUX). BMJ. 2013;346:1908–19.
6. Faria R, Bojke L, Epstein D, et al. Cost-effectiveness of laparoscopic fundoplication versus continued medical management for the treatment of gastro-oesophageal reflux disease based on long-term follow-up of the REFLUX trial. Br J Surg. 2013;100:1205–13.
7. Anvari M, Allen C, Marshall J, et al. A randomized controlled trial of laparoscopic Nissen fundoplication versus proton pump inhibitors for the treatment of patients with chronic gastro-esophageal reflux disease (GERD): 3-year outcomes. Surg Endosc. 2011;25:2547–54.
8. Lee Y, Tahir U, Tessier L, et al. Long-term outcomes following Dor, Toupet, and Nissen fundoplication: a network meta-analysis of randomized controlled trials. Surg Endosc. 2023;37:5052–64.
9. Cadière GB, Rajan A, Rquibate M, et al. Endoluminal fundoplication (ELF) – evolution of EsophyX™, a new surgical device for transoral surgery. Minim Invasive Ther Allied Technol. 2006;15:348–55.
10. Bell RC, Cadiere GB. Transoral rotational esophagogastric fundoplication: technical, anatomical, and safety considerations. Surg Endosc. 2011;25:2387–99.
11. Testoni PA, Mazzoleni G, Testoni SGG. Transoral incisionless fundoplication for gastro-esophageal reflux disease: techniques and outcomes. World J Gastrointest Pharmacol Ther. 2016;7:179–89.
12. Roy-Shapira A, Bapaye A, Date S, et al. Trans-oral anterior fundoplication: 5-year follow-up of pilot study. Surg Endosc. 2015;29:3717–21.
13. Testoni PA, Testoni S, Mazzoleni G, et al. Transoral incisionless fundoplication with an ultrasonic surgical endostapler for the treatment of gastro-esophageal reflux disease: 12-month outcomes. Endoscopy. 2020;52:469–73.
14. Weitzendorfer M, Spaun GO, Antoniou SA, et al. Clinical feasibility of a new full-thickness endoscopic plication device (GERDx™) for patients with GERD: results of a prospective trial. Surg Endosc. 2018;32:2541–9.
15. Inoue H, Ito H, Ikeda H, et al. Anti-reflux mucosectomy for gastroesophageal reflux disease in the absence of hiatus hernia: a pilot study. Ann Gastroenterol. 2014;27:346–51.
16. Inoue H, Tanabe M, de Santiago ER, et al. Antireflux mucosal ablation (ARMA) as a new treatment for gastroesophageal reflux refractory to proton pump inhibitors: a pilot study. Endosc Int Open. 2020;8:E133–8.
17. Triadafilopoulos G. Stretta: a valuable endoscopic treatment modality for gastroesophageal reflux disease. World J Gastroenterol. 2014;20:7730–8.
18. Perry KA, Banerjee A, Melvin WS. Radiofrequency energy delivery to the lower esophageal sphincter reduces esophageal acid exposure and improves GERD symptoms: a systematic review and meta-analysis. Surg Laparosc Endosc Percutan Tech. 2012;22:283–8.
19. Fass R, Cahn F, Scotti DJ, Gregory DA. Systematic review and meta-analysis of controlled and prospective cohort efficacy studies of endoscopic radiofrequency for treatment of gastro-esophageal reflux disease. Surg Endosc. 2017;31:4865–82.
20. Noar M, Squires P, Noar E, Lee M. Long-term maintenance effect of radiofrequency energy delivery for refractory GERD: a decade later. Surg Endosc. 2014;28:2323–33.

21. Lipka S, Kumar A, Richter JE. No evidence for efficacy of radiofrequency ablation for treatment of gastroesophageal reflux disease: a systematic review and meta-analysis. Clin Gastroenterol Hepatol. 2015;13:1058–67.
22. Huang X, Chen S, Zhao H, et al. Efficacy of transoral incisionless fundoplication (TIF) for the treatment of GERD: a systematic review with meta-analysis. Surg Endosc. 2017;31:1032–44.
23. McCarty TR, Itidiare M, Njei B, Rustagi T. Efficacy of transoral incisionless fundoplication for refractory gastroesophageal reflux disease: a systematic review and meta-analysis. Endoscopy. 2018;50:708–25.
24. Chandan S, Mohan BP, Khan SR, et al. Clinical efficacy and safety of magnetic sphincter augmentation (MSA) and transoral incisionless fundoplication (TIF2) in refractory gastroesophageal reflux disease (GERD): a systematic review and meta-analysis. Endosc Int Open. 2021;09:E583–98.
25. Testoni S, Hassan C, Mazzoleni G, et al. Long-term outcomes of transoral incisionless fundoplication for gastro-esophageal reflux disease: systematic-review and meta-analysis. Endosc Int Open. 2021;09:E239–46.
26. Ramai D, Shapiro A, Barakat M, et al. Adverse events associated with transoral incisionless fundoplication (TIF) for chronic gastroesophageal reflux disease: a MAUDE database analysis. Surg Endosc. 2022;36:4956–9.
27. Kim HJ, Kwon CI, Kessler W, et al. Long-term follow-up results of endoscopic treatment of gastroesophageal reflux disease with the MUSE™ endoscopic stapling device. Surg Endosc. 2016;30:3402–8.
28. Shen S, Yu G, Guo X, et al. The long-term efficacy of transoral incisionless fundoplication with Medigus Ultrasonic Surgical Endostapler (MUSE) for gastroesophageal reflux disease. Esophagus. 2023;20:581–6.
29. Testoni SGG, Cilona MB, Mazzoleni G, et al. Transoral incisionless fundoplication with Medigus ultrasonic surgical endostapler (MUSE) for the treatment of gastro-esophageal reflux disease: outcomes up to 3 years. Surg Endosc. 2022;36:5023–31.
30. Testoni SGG, Pantaleo G, Contu F, et al. Comparison of EsophyX2.0 and MUSE systems for transoral incisionless fundoplication: technical aspects and outcomes up to 3 years. Dig Endosc. 2024;36(11):1232–44.
31. Rausa E, Ferrari D, Kelly ME, et al. Efficacy of laparoscopic Toupet fundoplication compared to endoscopic and surgical procedures for GERD treatment: a randomized trials network meta-analysis. Langenbeck's Arch Surg. 2023;408:52–63.
32. Kalapala R, Karyampudi A, Nabi Z, et al. Endoscopic full-thickness plication for the treatment of PPI-dependent GERD: results from a randomised, sham controlled trial. Gut. 2022;71:686–94.
33. Rodríguez de Santiago E, Sanchez-Vegazo CT, Peñas B, et al. Antireflux mucosectomy (ARMS) and antireflux mucosal ablation (ARMA) for gastroesophageal reflux disease: a systematic review and meta-analysis. Endosc Int Open. 2021;9(11):E1740–51.

Open Access This chapter is licensed under the terms of the Creative Commons Attribution-NonCommercial 4.0 International License (http://creativecommons.org/licenses/by-nc/4.0/), which permits any noncommercial use, sharing, adaptation, distribution and reproduction in any medium or format, as long as you give appropriate credit to the original author(s) and the source, provide a link to the Creative Commons license and indicate if changes were made.

The images or other third party material in this chapter are included in the chapter's Creative Commons license, unless indicated otherwise in a credit line to the material. If material is not included in the chapter's Creative Commons license and your intended use is not permitted by statutory regulation or exceeds the permitted use, you will need to obtain permission directly from the copyright holder.

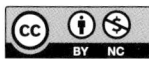

Hypotonic Lower Esophageal Sphincter and Hiatal Hernia: Clinical Symptoms and Diagnosis

Stefano Siboni and Marco Sozzi

7.1 Introduction

Hypotonic lower esophageal sphincter (LES) and hiatal hernia are two interrelated conditions that significantly contribute to gastroesophageal reflux disease (GERD). A comprehensive assessment of the clinical presentation and objective tests is essential for a confident GERD diagnosis and for an effective treatment. This chapter will explore the anatomical bases, pathophysiology, symptoms and diagnostic approaches of hypotonic LES and hiatal hernia.

7.2 Anatomy and Physiology

The LES, also called "intrinsic sphincter" constitutes a specialized region of the esophagogastric junction (EGJ) where smooth muscle maintains tonic contraction. This high-pressure zone typically extends 3–4 centimeters in length and generates a resting pressure between 10 and 30 mmHg. The pressure within the LES is influenced by several factors, including intra-abdominal pressure and neural control. A hypotonic LES is characterized by reduced pressure, which can lead to increased susceptibility to reflux. When the LES and the crural diaphragm (CD) (extrinsic sphincter) are superimposed, they work in synergy and create an effective barrier against backward reflux of gastric contents [1].

Hiatal hernia (HH) involves an anatomical disruption of the EGJ [2]. The condition is usually characterized by the displacement of the LES above the diaphragm, accompanied by a weakening of the phrenoesophageal ligament and a loss of the CD's contribution to the sphincter function. Four distinct types of HH exist, with

S. Siboni (✉) · M. Sozzi
General and Emergency Surgery, IRCCS Policlinico San Donato, San Donato Milanese, Italy
e-mail: stefano.siboni@grupposandonato.it; marcosozzi92@gmail.com

type I (sliding) representing approximately 95% of cases. The remaining types include pure paraesophageal (type II), mixed (type III), and complex (type IV) hernias, each with distinct anatomical features and clinical implications.

7.3 Clinical Presentation

Patients with hypotonic LES and HH typically present with a broad spectrum of symptoms. Heartburn and regurgitation are considered "typical symptoms" as they are often associated with a conclusive diagnosis of GERD. Chest or epigastric pain may also be present, even though they are not as specific as the typical symptoms. Finally, a higher rate of patients may experience extra-esophageal symptoms, such as cough or other respiratory symptoms (i.e., hoarseness, throat clearing), but the likelihood of correlation with pathologic reflux is low [3].

The clinical presentation and the burden of symptoms vary among the patients, ranging from asymptomatic to those who experience severe manifestations. The severity of symptoms can vary based on factors such as hernia size and LES function.

7.3.1 Alarming Symptoms

Certain clinical features warrant immediate attention and expedited evaluation. These warning signs include progressive dysphagia, painful swallowing (odynophagia), unintentional weight loss, gastrointestinal bleeding, and iron deficiency anemia. The presence of these features may indicate complications or alternative diagnoses requiring prompt investigation.

7.4 Diagnosis

7.4.1 Initial Assessment

One of the most crucial aspects of HH management is the first clinical assessment. Physicians should characterize the symptoms in detail, including their onset, progression, frequency, and severity. Given the important overlap of the symptoms with other conditions (i.e., functional heartburn, reflux hypersensitivity other gastrointestinal [GI] tract brain-gut interaction disorders), before escalation of medical treatment and, more importantly, before surgery, it is critical to obtain a definitive diagnosis. Even though internationally validated questionnaires exist, their accuracy in predicting pathologic GERD is low, having a sensitivity of 67% and a specificity of 65% [4].

7.4.2 Physical Examination

Physical examination, while often normal in uncomplicated cases, should include the calculation of the body mass index (BMI), waist circumference and general abdominal examination. Central obesity, in fact, is associated with an increased thoraco-abdominal gradient, HH and hypotonic LES [5, 6].

7.4.3 Upper Gastrointestinal Endoscopy

Upper-GI endoscopy plays a crucial role in the diagnostic process of patients with suspected GERD, since it provides a comprehensive visual examination of the esophagus, LES and stomach. There are several endoscopic definitive criteria for GERD according to the Lyon Consensus 2.0, in particular Los Angeles B, C or D esophagitis, peptic stricture and Barrett's esophagus [7].

Another important role of upper-GI endoscopy is the assessment of the EGJ in retroflexed view (Fig. 7.1).

The evaluation of EGJ integrity has evolved significantly since the initial Hill classification was introduced in 1996 [8]. This earlier method, based entirely upon the presence of the flap valve, suffered from significant drawbacks, including inconsistent standardization and terminology and difficulties in the distinction of grades.

Recognizing these limitations, the American Foregut Society (AFS) developed an innovative classification system [9]. This novel approach provides a more precise method to assess the EGJ integrity, by focusing on three critical elements: the axial length of the HH, the width of the hiatal opening, and the presence of the flap valve. By breaking down the assessment into these specific components, the AFS classification offers a more comprehensive and reproducible approach to understand EGJ structural integrity.

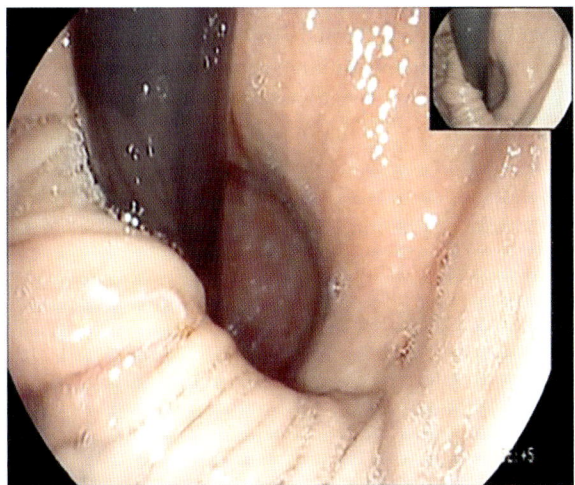

Fig. 7.1 Retroflexed endoscopic view of hiatal hernia

Table 7.1 Correlation between American Foregut Society grades and parameters of esophagogastric junction disruption at high-resolution manometry

	Grade I	Grade II	Grade III	Grade IV	p-value
EGJ contractile integral	60.0 ± 29.2	41.1 ± 23.6	40.1 ± 18.8	21.5 ± 13.9	0.015
Hiatal hernia	–	0.3 ± 0.6	1.0 ± 0.8	2.5 ± 2.9	0.032
LES total length	2.1 ± 0.2	1.9 ± 0.4	2.0 ± 0.5	1.8 ± 0.4	0.495
LES intra-abdominal length	1.2 ± 0.9	0.5 ± 0.6	0.6 ± 0.8	0.1 ± 0.3	0.016
LES basal pressure	39.5 ± 12.5	28.1 ± 13.3	21.1 ± 7.8	12.6 ± 8.5	0.003
Straight leg raise >11 mmHg	2/5 (40.0)	2/16 (12.5)	11/24 (45.8)	6/7 (85.7)	0.010

EGJ esophagogastric junction, *LES* lower esophageal sphincter

The new AFS classification addresses several key limitations of the previous Hill classification. Firstly, it introduces a more standardized protocol that ensures consistent patient categorization. Secondly, the new system eliminates the vagueness of the previous classification method by introducing objective measurements, specifically the axial length of the HH and hiatal diameter, providing a more comprehensive understanding of the anti-reflux barrier's components. A prospective study using high-resolution manometry (HRM) and multichannel intraluminal impedance pH study (MII-pH) demonstrated a stepwise increase of esophageal acid exposure time (AET) and worse HRM competency parameters at higher AFS grades [10] (Table 7.1).

The major limitation of the endoscopic assessment is the invasiveness of the test and overrating of the HH size, due to inflation of the stomach during the examination.

7.4.4 Swallow Study

The barium swallow study is an important test in the evaluation of HH as it provides a clear anatomical picture. Particularly in cases of large HH, this examination is particularly useful to assess the esophageal and gastric contour and to evaluate esophageal and gastric emptying, which may be affected in these patients. Specific diagnostic features include a "wide-open" gastroesophageal junction, retrograde barium flow, and potential retrocardiac air-fluid levels in cases of HH (Fig. 7.2).

While barium swallow is non-invasive and provides real-time swallowing dynamics, it has limitations. It cannot measure LES pressure directly and might miss small or subtle hernias. Therefore, it is typically used complementarily with other diagnostic tools like endoscopy, HRM, and pH monitoring to provide a comprehensive evaluation.

7.4.5 High-Resolution Manometry

HRM is a sophisticated diagnostic tool for evaluating LES function and anatomy, and is considered the gold standard for the diagnosis of HH [11]. Moreover, it

Fig. 7.2 Hiatal hernia at barium swallow study

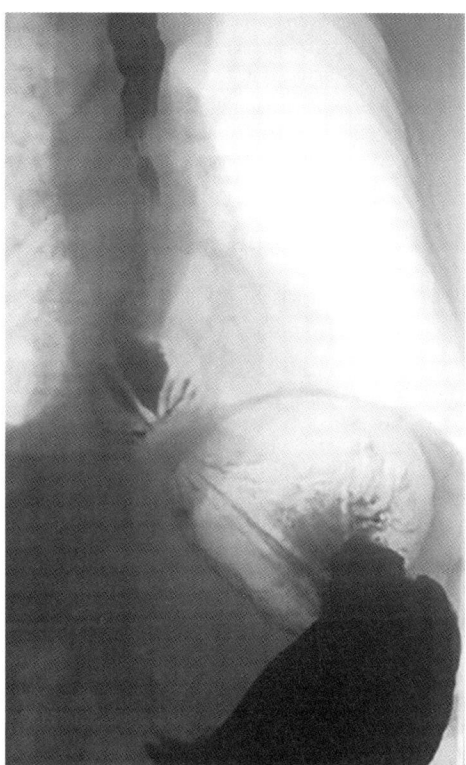

provides data on esophageal motility, and several provocative maneuvers can highlight a deficiency in contractile reserve (multiple rapid swallows) [12] or EGJ competency (straight leg raise maneuver) [13].

Key diagnostic parameters in defective LES include basal LES pressure and length (total and intra-abdominal). In 2014, Nicodeme et al. introduced the EGJ contractile integral, a high-resolution parameter that integrates EGJ length and pressure and is able to predict a pathologic AET better than LES basal pressure [14].

The Chicago Classification version 4.0 provides a precise classification of HH, segregating patients into type I (LES and CD superimposed), type II (LES-CD separation <3 cm) and type III (LES-CD separation >3 cm) [15].

Recently, the Milan score, a novel tool proposed to make GERD diagnosis more efficient, has been introduced and validated [16]. It integrates four HRM parameters (EGJ type, ineffective esophageal motility, EGJ contractile integral, and response to the straight leg raise maneuver), and it provides a comprehensive risk assessment of pathologic GERD (Fig. 7.3).

While HRM cannot independently diagnose GERD, it offers crucial information for surgical planning, helping to determine appropriate fundoplication techniques and predicting postoperative dysphagia risk.

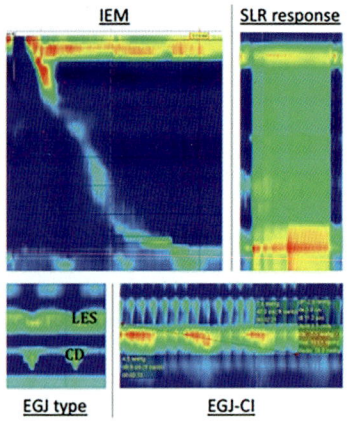

Fig. 7.3 Parameters related to gastroesophageal reflux disease included in the Milan score

CD, crural diaphragm; *EGJ*, esophagogastric junction; *EGJ-CI*, esophagogastric junction contractile integral; *IEM*, ineffective esophageal motility; *LES*, lower esophageal sphincter; *SLR*, straight leg raise.

7.4.6 Reflux Monitoring Test

Twenty-four-hour pH monitoring quantifies acid exposure and correlates symptoms with reflux events. This test generates several important parameters, including total AET, frequency of reflux episodes, and symptom correlation indices. The DeMeester score provides a composite measure of acid reflux severity [17].

Reflux monitoring tests are essential diagnostic tools for patients with HH, in order to provide a definitive GERD diagnosis defined as AET >6% according to the Lyon Consensus 2.0 [7].

The MII-pH represents an advanced diagnostic approach. Unlike traditional pH monitoring, this technique can detect both acid and non-acid reflux events. This capability is crucial for identifying non-acid reflux and to better correlate symptoms with reflux episodes.

A reliable alternative to MII-pH is the wireless 48- or 96-hour pH test, which is considered the gold standard for GERD diagnosis as it overcomes the day-to-day variability of the MII-pH and it allows a more real-life assessment of patients' daily activities.

7.4.7 Diagnostic Algorithm

For patients presenting with typical symptoms and no warning signs, an initial trial of empiric proton pump inhibitor (PPI) therapy is often appropriate, with response assessment after 4–8 weeks. However, the presence of warning signs mandates immediate endoscopic evaluation followed by additional testing based on initial findings. For patients presenting with atypical symptoms, the Lyon Consensus 2.0 warrants upfront pathophysiological tests in order to avoid PPI over-prescription [7]. In any case, in order to achieve a definitive diagnosis and correct assessment of a potential disruption of the EGJ, HRM and reflux monitoring tests are mandatory, after the execution of an index endoscopy.

7.5 Conclusion

Hypotonic LES and HH are conditions that contribute significantly to GERD symptoms and diagnosis. A thorough understanding of their clinical manifestations and available diagnostic techniques is crucial for effective management. Continued research is necessary to enhance treatment strategies and improve patient outcomes in those suffering from these gastrointestinal disorders.

References

1. Mittal RK, Fischer M, McCallum RW, et al. Human lower esophageal sphincter pressure response to increased intra-abdominal pressure. Am J Phys. 1990;258(4 Pt 1):G624–30.
2. Jones MP, Sloan SS, Rabine JC, et al. Hiatal hernia size is the dominant determinant of esophagitis presence and severity in gastroesophageal reflux disease. Am J Gastroenterol. 2001;96(6):1711–7.
3. Eusebi LH, Ratnakumaran R, Yuan Y, et al. Global prevalence of, and risk factors for, gastro-oesophageal reflux symptoms: a meta-analysis. Gut. 2018;67:430–40.
4. Simadibrata DM, Ngadiono E, Sinuraya FAG, et al. Diagnostic accuracy of gastroesophageal reflux disease questionnaire for gastroesophageal reflux disease: a systematic review and meta-analysis. Neurogastroenterol Motil. 2023;35(12):e14619.
5. Pandolfino JE, El-Serag HB, Zhang Q, et al. Obesity: a challenge to esophagogastric junction integrity. Gastroenterology. 2006;130(3):639–49.
6. Ayazi S, Hagen JA, Chan LS, et al. Obesity and gastroesophageal reflux: quantifying the association between body mass index, esophageal acid exposure, and lower esophageal sphincter status in a large series of patients with reflux symptoms. J Gastrointest Surg. 2009;13(8):1440–7.
7. Gyawali CP, Yadlapati R, Fass R, et al. Updates to the modern diagnosis of GERD: Lyon consensus 2.0. Gut. 2024;73(2):361–71.
8. Hill LD, Kozarek RA, Kraemer SJ, et al. The gastro- esophageal flap valve: in vitro and in vivo observations. Gastrointest Endosc. 1996;44:541–7.
9. Nguyen NT, Thosani NC, Canto MI, et al. The American Foregut Society white paper on the endoscopic classification of esophagogastric junction integrity. Foregut. 2022;2(4):263451612211269.
10. Siboni S, Sozzi M, Kersik A, et al. Does the American Foregut Society endoscopic classification of esophago-gastric junction integrity predict acid reflux and esophago-gastric junction disruption? Foregut. 2024. https://doi.org/10.1177/26345161241230940.
11. Tolone S, Savarino E, Zaninotto G, et al. High-resolution manometry is superior to endoscopy and radiology in assessing and grading sliding hiatal hernia: a comparison with surgical in vivo evaluation. United European Gastroenterol J. 2018;6(7):981–9.
12. Fox MR, Sweis R, Yadlapati R, et al. Chicago classification version 4.0© technical review: update on standard high-resolution manometry protocol for the assessment of esophageal motility. Neurogastroenterol Motil. 2021;33(4):e14120.
13. Siboni S, Kristo I, Rogers BD, et al. Improving the diagnostic yield of high-resolution esophageal manometry for GERD: the "Straight Leg-Raise" international study. Clin Gastroenterol Hepatol. 2023;21(7):1761–70.e1.
14. Nicodème F, Pipa-Muniz M, Khanna K, et al. Quantifying esophagogastric junction contractility with a novel HRM topographic metric, the EGJ-contractile integral: normative values and preliminary evaluation in PPI non-responders. Neurogastroenterol Motil. 2014;26(3):353–60.

15. Yadlapati R, Kahrilas PJ, Fox MR, et al. Esophageal motility disorders on high-resolution manometry: Chicago classification version 4.0©. Neurogastroenterol Motil. 2021;33(1):e14058.
16. Siboni S, Sozzi M, Kristo I, et al. The Milan score: a novel manometric tool for a more efficient diagnosis of gastro-esophageal reflux disease. United European Gastroenterol J. 2024;12(5):552–61.
17. Johnson LF, Demeester TR. Twenty-four-hour pH monitoring of the distal esophagus. A quantitative measure of gastroesophageal reflux. Am J Gastroenterol. 1974;62(4):325–32.

Open Access This chapter is licensed under the terms of the Creative Commons Attribution-NonCommercial 4.0 International License (http://creativecommons.org/licenses/by-nc/4.0/), which permits any noncommercial use, sharing, adaptation, distribution and reproduction in any medium or format, as long as you give appropriate credit to the original author(s) and the source, provide a link to the Creative Commons license and indicate if changes were made.

The images or other third party material in this chapter are included in the chapter's Creative Commons license, unless indicated otherwise in a credit line to the material. If material is not included in the chapter's Creative Commons license and your intended use is not permitted by statutory regulation or exceeds the permitted use, you will need to obtain permission directly from the copyright holder.

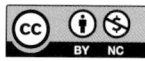

Neuromuscular Diagnosis by Esophageal Tests

8

Pierfrancesco Visaggi

8.1 Introduction

Swallowing is a complex, coordinated process divided into four phases: oral preparatory, oral propulsive, pharyngeal, and esophageal. The oral preparatory phase, which is voluntary, includes actions such as biting, lip closure, and chewing. In the oral propulsive phase, the tongue pushes the bolus against the palate, moving it from the mouth to the pharynx. The pharyngeal phase, which occurs automatically and involuntarily, transfers the bolus from the pharynx to the esophagus. Lastly, the esophageal phase moves the bolus down the esophagus to the stomach. Oropharyngeal dysphagia refers to any dysfunction in the oral preparatory, propulsive, or pharyngeal phases, leading to challenges in moving food or liquid from the mouth to the esophagus [1]. A variety of systemic diseases can cause oropharyngeal dysphagia by means of neuromuscular loss of function. Neuromuscular, rheumatologic, immunologic, and endocrinologic disorders can impair the oropharyngeal phase of swallowing. These conditions affect the swallowing process in distinct ways, leading to considerable clinical challenges and necessitating individualized diagnostic and management approaches.

The prevalence of oropharyngeal dysphagia varies according to the target population. Elderly patients and patients with neurological or neurodegenerative diseases have the highest prevalence [2]. Regardless of the etiology, individuals with oropharyngeal dysphagia may report a range of digestive and respiratory symptoms. Common symptoms include coughing or choking while eating or drinking, fear related to eating, changes in voice quality (often

---

P. Visaggi (✉)
Department of Translational Research and New Technologies in Medicine and Surgery, University of Pisa, Pisa, Italy
e-mail: pierfrancesco.visaggi@phd.unipi.it

sounding wet or gurgly) during meals, sensations of food being lodged in the throat, feeling of residual food in the pharynx, prolonged meal times, meal-related fatigue, dietary limitations to specific textures, and decreased enjoyment of eating [3, 4]. Accordingly, indicators of oropharyngeal dysphagia can be categorized into those that signify compromised swallowing safety and those that reflect decreased swallowing efficiency. Signs of safety impairment are associated with airway penetration and aspiration, while efficiency-related signs include prolonged oral or pharyngeal phases, anterior bolus leakage due to weak labial seal, premature bolus entry into the pharynx, piecemeal swallowing, nasal regurgitation, and oral or pharyngeal residue [5].

8.2 Etiology of Neuromuscolar Dysphagia

8.2.1 Neurologic and Neuromuscular Disorders

Oropharyngeal dysphagia can derive from neuromuscular diseases. The most common causes include multiple sclerosis, Parkinson's disease, and amyotrophic lateral sclerosis. Additionally, disorders such as myasthenia gravis and polymyositis/dermatomyositis particularly impact the oropharyngeal area by weakening muscles and disrupting coordination. Finally, post-stroke dysphagia represents a major cause of oropharyngeal dysphagia, especially in the elderly [2].

8.2.2 Rheumatologic and Immunologic Disorders

Systemic sclerosis, Sjogren's syndrome, systemic lupus erythematosus, and connective tissue diseases can cause oropharyngeal dysphagia due to impaired neuromuscular function and subsequent esophageal dysmotility. Similarly, immunologic disorders like pemphigus and sarcoidosis can impact both esophageal and oropharyngeal areas, through mucosal involvement and granulomatous inflammation, respectively [6]. Immune-mediated esophageal inflammation, such as eosinophilic esophagitis and lymphocytic esophagitis, can also lead to dysphagia by means of neuromuscular involvement with loss of function [7, 8].

8.2.3 Endocrine Disorders

Diabetes mellitus and hypothyroidism can also lead to dysphagia. In the case of diabetes, autonomic neuropathy may hinder esophageal motility, whereas hypothyroidism can result in muscle weakness and reduced gastrointestinal motility, impacting both the esophageal and oropharyngeal phases of swallowing [9].

8.3 Diagnosis of Neuromuscolar Dysphagia

Careful clinical history taking can help suspecting oropharyngeal dysphagia, although symptoms alone are insufficient to reach a conclusive diagnosis [10]. In particular, difficulty in initiating swallowing, post-deglutitive cough, nasal regurgitation, aspiration, choking, and repetitive swallowing are suggestive of oropharyngeal dysphagia. Of note, the presence of "high dysphagia", that is, the feeling of food bolus getting stuck up in the throat, is not specific for oropharyngeal dysphagia. In this regard, patients with lower esophageal strictures frequently report perceiving the bolus sticking in the neck even in the absence of proximal esophageal abnormalities [11, 12]. Accordingly, when patients localize dysphagia to the sternal notch or the throat, this is unreliable [13].

Instrumental assessment of oropharyngeal dysphagia can help identify the underlying cause of symptoms. Available diagnostic strategies include the volume-viscosity swallow test (V-VST), the fiberoptic endoscopic evaluation of swallowing (FEES), videofluoroscopic swallowing study (VFSS), and high-resolution pharyngeal manometry (HRPM).

The V-VST is a clinical tool that aids in the preliminary diagnosis of swallowing disorders. It helps to pinpoint patients who may need more detailed assessments and guides treatment options for individuals who are not candidates for VFS or FEES.

FEES is a key procedure for assessing swallowing function, focusing on the pharynx, tongue base, and larynx's anatomy and movement. FEES is recognized as a gold standard technique for evaluating the physiology and functionality of swallowing, especially in patients with oropharyngeal dysphagia. It is a low-risk procedure with minimal complications and can be effectively administered in various settings, including patients with limited positioning abilities. Indications for FEES include typical signs and symptoms of oropharyngeal dysphagia, such as prolonged meal times, difficulty handling saliva, or medication-related dysphagia. The procedure also aids in selecting appropriate dietary modifications, creating tailored treatment approaches, and monitoring the effectiveness of interventions and disease progression. Of note, FEES is contraindicated in patients with complete bilateral nasal obstruction, respiratory rates over 35 breaths per minute, diminished consciousness, or those who decline oral intake [14]. Similar to FEES, VFS represents another key examination for the assessment of oropharyngeal dysphagia. The study consists in a dynamic evaluation of the swallow function by means of a contrast-enriched bolus administered during radiological recording [15].

HRPM is a catheter-based assessment method that allows the evaluation of pharyngeal and upper esophageal sphincter motor function. The first consensus on the protocol and relevant metrics of HRPM was developed only recently. The authors categorized 22 HRPM-impedance metrics into three classes: pharyngeal lumen occlusive pressures, hypopharyngeal intrabolus pressures, and upper esophageal sphincter function. However, only eight HRPM-impedance metrics achieved consensus agreement: pharyngeal contractile integral (CI), velopharyngeal CI, hypopharyngeal CI, hypopharyngeal pressure at nadir impedance, upper esophageal sphincter integrated relaxation pressure, relaxation time, and maximum admittance

[16]. HRPM offers unique advantages over other instrumental methods, such as FEES and VFSS, by providing detailed measurements of motor functions associated with swallowing inefficiency (e.g., residue) or safety concerns (e.g., aspiration or penetration) identified in FEES and/or VFSS. HRM enables precise assessment of pharyngeal contractility, upper esophageal sphincter relaxation, and bolus pressurization. Accordingly, especially patients whose pharyngeal contractility and upper esophageal sphincter functions are unclear may benefit most from HRPM [16].

References

1. Clavé P, Shaker R. Dysphagia: current reality and scope of the problem. Nat Rev Gastroenterol Hepatol. 2015;12(5):259–70.
2. Clavé P, Rofes L, Carrión S, et al. Pathophysiology, relevance and natural history of oropharyngeal dysphagia among older people. Nestle Nutr Inst Workshop Ser. 2012;72:57–66.
3. Shaheen H, Adeel H. Oropharyngeal dysphagia. In: Ujiki MB, Hedberg HM, editors. Dysphagia. 1st ed. Academic Press; 2024. p. 1–39.
4. Yang S, Park JW, et al. Clinical practice guidelines for oropharyngeal dysphagia. Ann Rehabil Med. 2023;47(Suppl 1):S1–S26.
5. Namasivayam-MacDonald AM, Riquelme LF. Presbyphagia to dysphagia: multiple perspectives and strategies for quality care of older adults. Semin Speech Lang. 2019;40(3):227–42.
6. Reddy CA, McGowan E, Yadlapati R, Peterson K. AGA clinical practice update on esophageal dysfunction due to disordered immunity and infection: expert review. Clin Gastroenterol Hepatol. 2024;22(12):2378–87.
7. Visaggi P, Ghisa M, Barberio B, et al. Systematic review: esophageal motility patterns in patients with eosinophilic esophagitis. Dig Liver Dis. 2022;54(9):1143–52.
8. Visaggi P, Savarino E, Del Corso G, et al. Clinical characteristics, endoscopic findings, and treatment outcomes in lymphocytic esophagitis compared with eosinophilic esophagitis. Am J Gastroenterol. 2025;120(2):469–72.
9. Krishnan B, Babu S, Walker J, et al. Gastrointestinal complications of diabetes mellitus. World J Diabetes. 2013;4(3):51–63.
10. Malagelada JR, Bazzoli F, Boeckxstaens G, et al. World gastroenterology organisation global guidelines: dysphagia—global guidelines and cascades update September 2014. J Clin Gastroenterol. 2015;49(5):370–8.
11. Smith JK, Matheus MG, Castillo M. Imaging manifestations of neurosarcoidosis. AJR Am J Roentgenol. 2004;182(2):289–95.
12. Wilcox CM, Alexander LN, Clark WS. Localization of an obstructing esophageal lesion. Is the patient accurate? Dig Dis Sci. 1995;40(10):2192–6.
13. Liu LWC, Andrews CN, Armstrong D, et al. Clinical practice guidelines for the assessment of uninvestigated esophageal dysphagia. J Can Assoc Gastroenterol. 2018;1(1):5–19.
14. Schindler A, Baijens LWJ, Geneid A, Pizzorni N. Phoniatricians and otorhinolaryngologists approaching oropharyngeal dysphagia: an update on FEES. Eur Arch Otorrinolaringol. 2022;279(6):2727–42.
15. Labeit B, Michou E, Hamdy S, et al. The assessment of dysphagia after stroke: state of the art and future directions. Lancet Neurol. 2023;22(9):858–70.
16. Omari TI, Ciucci M, Gozdzikowska K, et al. High-resolution pharyngeal manometry and impedance: protocols and metrics-recommendations of a High-Resolution Pharyngeal Manometry International Working Group. Dysphagia. 2020;35(2):281–95.

Open Access This chapter is licensed under the terms of the Creative Commons Attribution-NonCommercial 4.0 International License (http://creativecommons.org/licenses/by-nc/4.0/), which permits any noncommercial use, sharing, adaptation, distribution and reproduction in any medium or format, as long as you give appropriate credit to the original author(s) and the source, provide a link to the Creative Commons license and indicate if changes were made.

The images or other third party material in this chapter are included in the chapter's Creative Commons license, unless indicated otherwise in a credit line to the material. If material is not included in the chapter's Creative Commons license and your intended use is not permitted by statutory regulation or exceeds the permitted use, you will need to obtain permission directly from the copyright holder.

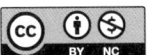

Esophagitis and Barrett's Esophagus

Giuseppe Galloro, Rosa Maione, and Alessia Chini

9.1 Esophagitis

9.1.1 Introduction

Esophagitis refers to inflammation or damage to the esophageal mucosa due to a variety of physical, chemical and infectious agents. The most common cause of esophagitis is gastroesophageal reflux disease, in which the frequent reflux of gastric content into the esophagus leads to mucosal injury; other causes include radiation, infections, medications, and eosinophilic and lymphocytic esophagitis [1]. Some of these conditions present with nonspecific lesions and a clinic-pathological correlation is required for diagnosis, while others show typical histological characteristics which enable the pathologist to reach the diagnosis.

Although there are many etiologies of esophagitis, the clinical presentation is essentially similar and includes retrosternal chest pain, dysphagia, odynophagia, and heartburn [2].

9.1.2 Reflux Esophagitis

Gastroesophageal reflux disease (GERD) is a very common disorder, with a widely variable global prevalence of 8–33%; it can affect patients of all ages and can present with a wide variety of symptoms, such as regurgitation, heartburn, dysphagia and extra-esophageal manifestations (asthma, hoarseness, chronic cough) [1, 3]. Several factors may predispose patients to GERD: hiatal hernia, reduced lower esophageal sphincter tone, gastric hypersecretory states, delayed gastric emptying

---

G. Galloro (✉) · R. Maione · A. Chini
Digestive Surgical Endoscopy Unit, Department of Clinical Medicine and Surgery, University of Naples Federico II – School of Medicine, Naples, Italy
e-mail: giuseppe.galloro@unina.it; rosamaione95@libero.it; dr.alessiachini@gmail.com

and loss of esophageal peristaltic function. In some cases, gastroesophageal reflux is physiological, for example the brief reflux episodes that occur post-prandially but do not cause mucosal damage; pathological gastroesophageal reflux occurs when gastric and duodenal acid contents overwhelm the normal protective antireflux barriers and cause injuries to the esophageal mucosa [4]. The severity of esophagitis is closely correlated with the frequency and duration of acid exposure; at endoscopy, about 40% of patients have erosive esophagitis, characterized by erosions and ulcers in the distal esophagus, while the remaining patients have nonspecific endoscopic findings, such as erythema, edema and friability of the distal esophagus [5, 6]. Endoscopic biopsies may be helpful to confirm the presence of esophagitis and possible Barrett's esophagus, which occurs in 7–10% of patients [7]. The aim of treatment is improvement of symptoms, healing of erosive disease and prevention of long-term complications such as anemia, strictures, Barrett's esophagus, dysplasia and adenocarcinoma [2].

9.1.3 Eosinophilic Esophagitis

Eosinophilic esophagitis (EoE) is a primary, local immune-mediated disorder of the esophagus where esophageal symptoms are associated with an increased number of intraepithelial eosinophils at histopathological examination [8]. The pathogenesis of EoE is incompletely defined, but its incidence and prevalence are increasing worldwide. Probably, this is due to increased awareness and recognition among clinicians and pathologists of this disorder, which may have previously been under-recognized and misdiagnosed as GERD [2]. EoE is generally accepted to be induced by antigen sensitization especially through food, but also through environmental allergens. The inflammation is fairly organ specific because the antigens in eosinophilic esophagitis do not cause eosinophilic inflammation elsewhere in the gastrointestinal tract but only in the esophagus. EoE is not caused by acid reflux, even though the two can occur together, because of the high frequency of GERD. EoE is not manifested through the typical allergic pathway of IgE but is a local IgG4-mediated mucosal inflammation in the esophagus that leads to pathological changes in the entire esophageal wall, with submucosal fibrosis, remodelling and narrowing [9]. Clinical presentation varies with age and EoE is most common in male patients between 20 and 40 years. The typical symptom of EoE is dysphagia for solids, and it may be reported as a feeling of food moving slowly or as a feeling of food sticking in the chest for a long time after swallowing; in most cases, patients present to the emergency department when the food bolus has been stuck for hours. Other symptoms are regurgitation, vomiting, abdominal pain and failure to thrive, and many patients have a personal history of allergic asthma, food and environmental allergies.

A challenge for clinicians is to distinguish EoE from other upper gastrointestinal conditions: endoscopy can be helpful for the diagnosis, but the gold standard remains the histopathological examination of biopsy specimens, which requires six biopsies from multiple areas, either taken from sites of clear endoscopic abnormality, or two in the upper, two in the middle and two in the lower end of the esophagus

[9, 10]. The finding of >15 intraepithelial eosinophils/high power field (HPF) in one or more esophageal mucosal biopsy specimens is diagnostic of EoE [8]. Typical endoscopic features include concentric mucosal rings, which appear quite fixed and can lead to a trachealization of the esophagus, linear furrows extending through much of the lumen, white plaques, focal strictures, generalized edema and narrow esophagus. Therapeutic options include a dietary approach excluding dairy products, eggs, wheat, soy, peanut/tree nuts, fish/shellfish, legumes [11], medications, such as topical steroid therapy using orodispersible budesonide [12] or proton-pump inhibitors, or therapeutic endoscopic dilatation [13].

9.1.4 Lymphocytic Esophagitis

Lymphocytic esophagitis (LE) has only recently been described and is a rare esophageal condition characterized by an increased number of lymphocytes only in the epithelium of esophagus. This condition still represents an enigma, because the diagnostic criteria and clinical characteristics remain uncertain, and it is unclear whether it represents a manifestation of another disorder or a distinct clinical condition [14]. Data reported in the literature suggested that LE may be an allergic disorder due to an allergic or hypersensitivity reaction [15] or related to EoE or reflux esophagitis spectrum [16]. As in EoE, endoscopy with biopsy is mandatory and the gold standard for diagnosis is the histological examination showing an increased number of intraepithelial lymphocytes especially in the distal esophageal epithelium, but the exact number of lymphocytes required for the diagnosis has not been well defined (most commonly >50 lymphocytes per HPF) [14]. Patients with LE frequently report dysphagia, GERD-like symptoms and esophageal motility abnormalities; treatment options for LE are limited and are similar to those for EoE, including use of proton-pump inhibitors, swallowed topical steroids and endoscopic dilatation [17].

9.1.5 Infective Esophagitis

Infective esophagitis can be caused by bacteria, viruses, fungal and parasitic microorganisms, especially in immunocompromised patients. *Candida albicans* is the most common cause of infective esophagitis; it is a normal component of the normal flora of the gastrointestinal tract, but it can lead to inflammation in particular cases, especially in patients treated with antibiotics, corticosteroids or acid-suppressive therapy and in those affected by immunodeficiency syndromes or malignant neoplasms, while it is rarely described in immunocompetent patients [18, 19]. Oropharyngeal and esophageal candidiasis may be the first presentation of a disseminated disease. Endoscopy with brushing and biopsies is the most sensitive and specific method for diagnosis, showing focal or confluent patchy and whitish plaques overlying friable and erythematous mucosa, associated with ulcerations in severe cases. Although these findings are highly suggestive of candidiasis, they are not specific and not always present; the diagnosis is defined by histopathology, showing active esophagitis with budding spores, ulcer slough and fibrinopurulent exudate, with a frequent invasion of mucosal and submucosal blood vessels [2]. Herpes simplex virus (HSV) is the most common cause of viral esophagitis, occurring in patients who underwent solid organ or bone marrow transplantation or with immunodeficiency syndromes, and only occasionally in patients with normal immune function.

Endoscopic findings include nonspecific erosive esophagitis and focal or confluent superficial ulcerations with exudate, confirmed by histopathological examination. If HSV is suspected, tissue can be sent for viral culture to confirm the diagnosis and identify HSV resistant to acyclovir [20]. Cytomegalovirus, Epstein-Barr virus and varicella-zoster virus are other viral causes of infective esophagitis [2].

9.1.6 Pill Esophagitis

Pill esophagitis (PE) can be caused by some medications, whose caustic components can lead to mucosal injury if they have prolonged contact with the esophageal mucosa and dissolve in the esophagus; the most commonly implicated medications are antibiotics (tetracyclines and doxycycline), nonsteroidal anti-inflammatory drugs, bisphosphonates, ascorbic acid and iron supplements [21]. PE is more common in elderly patients, in those who have a lumen reduction which makes swallowing difficult, and those who take pills when lying down. The diagnosis is performed with endoscopy, showing single or multiple ulcers with different degrees of penetration, surrounded by regular mucosa [2].

9.1.7 Radiation Esophagitis

Radiation esophagitis (RE) derives from treatment with radiotherapy, especially for lung, esophageal, mediastinal and thoracic tumors, and the risk increases if patient is undergoing chemotherapy at the same time. RE usually occurs 2–3 weeks after the start of the radiotherapy and endoscopy shows mucositis and ulceration [22].

9.2 Barrett's Esophagus

9.2.1 Introduction

Barrett's esophagus (BE) is defined as a metaplastic conversion of the distal normal esophageal squamous mucosa (for at least 1 cm above the gastroesophageal junction) to intestinal columnar epithelium. This condition, developing in 5–15% of patients with chronic reflux symptoms undergoing upper endoscopy, is a complication of untreated long-term GERD, because chronic acid exposure damages the esophageal squamous cells, causing their replacement with mucus-secreting cells [23].

Factors associated with an increased risk of BE are male sex, age >50 years old, weight gain with abdominal adiposity, hiatal hernia. It is essential to recognize BE as it is a precancerous condition, representing the main risk factor for the onset of esophageal adenocarcinoma [24].

The transition from intestinal metaplasia to carcinoma is a multi-step process, during which cell modifications occur, resulting in the development of low-grade and high-grade dysplasia [25].

Endoscopic eradication of dysplasia is recommended by all international guidelines for patients with high-grade dysplasia (HGD) due to the high risk of progression to adenocarcinoma. On the other hand, the management of low-grade dysplasia (LGD) in BE remains controversial due to its overdiagnosis and variable risk of progression.

9.2.2 Diagnosis

The gold standard for BE diagnosis is endoscopy. On esophagogastroduodenoscopy it appears as a salmon-colored mucosa extending more than 1 cm proximal to the gastroesophageal junction. Many optical methods can help to detect the metaplastic mucosa, although a firm diagnosis is achieved by the histological examination of mucosal biopsies. During endoscopy, BE is defined using the Prague classification, based on circumferential (C) and maximum (M) extent from the gastroesophageal junction of metaplastic mucosa [26].

The histological diagnosis must be confirmed by a standardized bioptic sampling according to the Seattle Protocol, which involves 4-quadrant biopsy sampling every 2 cm throughout the entire length of the metaplastic esophageal mucosa. Furthermore, every mucosal irregularity should be sampled because in these areas it is more probable to find dysplastic tissue [27].

A high-quality endoscopic examination is a critical step for the diagnosis of BE; advanced endoscopic imaging provides enhancement of suspicious areas of metaplasia, guiding the biopsy sampling. Among the most innovative techniques, chromoendoscopy, virtual chromoendoscopy, confocal endomicroscopy and artificial intelligence are used. To enhance the atypical features of dysplastic mucosa, conventional chromoendoscopy involves applying dyes topically through a spray catheter, similar to what happens in white-light endoscopy. Methylene blue is the dye commonly used to detect BE because it is selectively absorbed by intestinal cells, whereas indigo carmine is not absorbed by cells, but its use highlights the mucosal irregularities, allowing BE identification. Acetic acid, a weak acid used as a nonabsorbed contrast agent, causes an acetowhitening reaction on the esophageal mucosa, which is followed by a focal redness in dysplastic BE; this event is defined by Longcroft-Wheaton et al. as a predictor of pre-neoplastic lesion [28].

The advancement of digital endoscopy has resulted in the development of virtual chromoendoscopy, an advanced imaging technique that allows the endoscopist to improve the visualization of the BE by using specific wavelengths of light (Fig. 9.1).

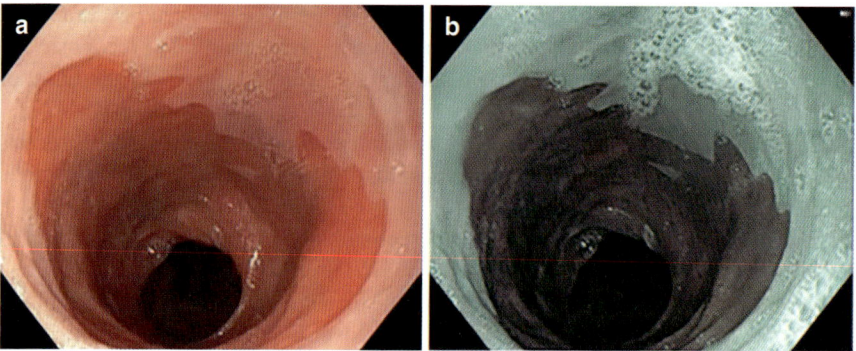

Fig. 9.1 Endoscopic evaluation of circumferential Barrett's esophagus (**a**) with white-light endoscopy and (**b**) narrow-band imaging

Narrow-band imaging (NBI) utilizes green and blue light to enhance superficial mucosal features like vascular patterns and mucosal irregularities without the need for contrast agents.

9.2.3 Management

It is difficult to predict the natural progression from the histological diagnosis of intestinal metaplasia to LGD and HGD and their neoplastic and clinical outcomes. The first step for the best management of dysplastic BE is histological confirmation of dysplasia; several studies showed that among patients with a histological diagnosis of LGD at the first endoscopic examination, dysplasia was not confirmed in 75% of cases on subsequent histological evaluations [29].

Failure to confirm LGD during surveillance can be explained by the similar cytologic features between inflammation-mediated injury and dysplasia, which makes it difficult to differentiate these two conditions and leads to an overdiagnosis of LGD; therefore, it was concluded that confirmation by two or more expert pathologists is necessary to increase the reliability of the histological diagnosis of LGD. A confirmed diagnosis of LGD involves a significant risk of neoplastic incidence, with a progression rate to HGD and esophageal adenocarcinoma from 0.5% to 13% per year [30].

Whereas for HGD there is consensus on the indication for eradication therapy, currently there is no widely approved management for LGD. For instance, the European Society of Gastrointestinal Endoscopy (ESGE) guidelines suggest that endoscopic eradication of LGD should be offered to patients with a confirmed histological diagnosis after a surveillance interval of six months [31]. Similarly, the latest guidelines from the American Society for Gastrointestinal Endoscopy (ASGE) and American Gastroenterological Association (AGA) recommend endoscopic eradication of LGD as a viable option for patients who have been diagnosed with LGD during a second examination within 3 to 6 months, even if both eradication therapy and surveillance are required [32, 33]. The histopathologic assessment of LGD in Japan differs from Western countries because it is defined as well-differentiated adenocarcinoma with low-grade atypia and noninvasive. In the current state, the Japan Gastroenterological Endoscopy Society (JGES) guidelines suggest endoscopic resection for HGD, while it is preferred to have 6-monthly endoscopic surveillance for LGD conditions [34].

9.2.4 Treatment

The first-line treatment of dysplastic BE should be endoscopic eradication therapy. Endoscopic eradication of dysplastic BE can be achieved by using different endoscopic techniques, including resective treatments such as endoscopic mucosal resection (EMR) and endoscopic submucosal dissection (ESD), and ablative treatments such as radiofrequency ablation (RFA), cryotherapy ablation and argon plasma coagulation (APC), or a combination of these techniques. The choice of therapeutic approach is based on the appearance of the esophageal mucosa affected by dysplasia. Ablative treatments, and mainly RFA, are preferred to treat flat BE dysplasia, while nodular BE should be treated with EMR or ESD [35].

EMR and ESD are endoscopic techniques performed for the treatment of nodular lesions of the esophageal mucosa. EMR is performed making an endoscopic snare resection of the flat mucosal lesion preceded by injection of a saline solution into the submucosal layer to lift the lesion area away from the deeper muscular layer. Konda et al. [36] demonstrated a rate of 95.9% for complete remission of dysplasia, with a recurrence of 8.1% after 33 months of follow-up. The most common complications of endoscopic resection performed for BE treatment is stricture, followed by bleeding and perforation. ESD is an advanced resective technique, more selective and requiring a higher level of expertise compared to EMR; furthermore, ESD has a higher complication rate.

Endoscopic resection has the advantage of allowing a histological examination of the resected specimen, which can determine the grade of dysplasia and the appropriate treatment; however, these procedures are characterized by a longer operative time and a higher complication rate compared to ablative endoscopic treatment.

The most frequently used ablative treatment is RFA, which is an endoscopic technique utilizing thermal energy to cause necrosis of dysplastic mucosa in the esophageal dysplastic mucosa and regeneration. This system consists of an energy generator, which is a bipolar electrode array with 60 tightly spaced electrodes encircling the balloon catheters. RFA can be performed with two different ablation devices, for focal or circumferential ablation. The circumferential balloon (HALO 360) is indicated for long-segment and circumferential BE, while the focal balloon (HALO 90) works better for focal lesions with a difficult anatomical localization, as with a hiatal hernia. The efficacy and safety of RFA are proven, even though recurrence after this ablative endoscopic treatment is possible: the annual rate of recurrence of BE after RFA is 5–8%, so patients treated with RFA should be closely followed up [37].

An emerging, alternative technique to radiofrequency is cryotherapy ablation, which uses a cryogen (liquid nitrogen or carbon dioxide) to rapidly cool the esophageal dysplastic mucosa, causing tissue necrosis, unlike RFA which uses heat energy.

This technique is noncontact and more focused than RFA, which may be why it has a lower risk of stricture incidence than RFA. In addition, cryotherapy can ablate deeper into the submucosa [38].

APC is a technique that uses a probe-based catheter with jet ionized argon gas to induce dysplastic tissue necrosis. Despite its effectiveness in the gastrointestinal tract and for BE treatment, this technique is susceptible to perforation of the esophageal mucosa. This has led to the creation of Hybrid-APC, an advanced form of this ablative technique that incorporates APC with a preventive submucosal injection [39].

References

1. Iwakiri K, Fujiwara Y, Manabe N, et al. Evidence-based clinical practice guidelines for gastroesophageal reflux disease 2021. J Gastroenterol. 2022;57:267–85.
2. Maguire A, Sheahan K. Pathology of esophagitis. Histopathology. 2012;60:864–79.
3. Gyawali CP, Kahrilas PJ, Savarino E, et al. Modern diagnosis of GERD: the Lyon consensus. Gut. 2018;67:1351–62.
4. Kahrilas PJ. Clinical practice. Gastro-esophageal reflux disease. N Engl J Med. 2008;359:1700–7.
5. Zagari RM, Fuccio L, Wallander MA, et al. Gastro-esophageal reflux symptoms, esophagitis and Barrett's esophagus in the general population: the Loiano-Monghidoro study. Gut. 2008;57:1354–9.
6. Dent J. Microscopic esophageal mucosal injury in nonerosive reflux disease. Clin Gastroenterol Hepatol. 2007;5:4–16.
7. Gilani N, Gerkin RD, Ramirez FC, et al. Prevalence of Barrett's esophagus in patients with moderate to severe erosive esophagitis. World J Gastroenterol. 2008;14:3518–22.
8. Furuta GT, Liacouros CA, Collins MH, et al. Eosiniphilic esophagitis in children and adults: a systematic review and consensus recommendations for diagnosis and treatment. Gastroenterology. 2007;133:1342–63.
9. Attwood SE. Overview of eosinophilic esophagitis. Br J Hosp Med (Lond). 2019;80:132–8.
10. Nielsen JA, Lager DJ, Lewin M, et al. The optimal number of biopsy fragments to establish a morphologic diagnosis of eosinophilic esophagitis. Am J Gastroenterol. 2014;109:515–20.
11. Gonsalves N, Yang GY, Doerfler B, et al. Elimination diet effectively treats eosinophilic esophagitis in adults; food reintroduction identifies causative factors. Gastroenterology. 2012;142:1451–9.
12. Miehlke S, Hruz P, Vieth M, et al. A randomised, double-blind trial comparing budesonide formulations and dosages for short-term treatment of eosinophilic esophagitis. Gut. 2016;65:390–9.
13. Schoepfer AM, Gonsalves N, Bussmann C, et al. Esophageal dilatation in eosinophilic esophagitis: effectiveness, safety and impact on the underlying inflammation. Am J Gastroenterol. 2010;105:1062–70.
14. Nguyen AD, Dunbar KB. How to approach lymphocytic esophagitis. Curr Gastroenterol Rep. 2017;19:24.
15. Zhang Z, Jain D, Brand M. Ringed esophagus secondary to lymphocytic esophagitis. Gastroenterol Hepatol. 2016;12:237–9.
16. Genta RM. Lymphocytic esophagitis. Gastroenterol Hepatol. 2015;11:559–61.

17. Haque S, Genta RM. Lymphocytic esophagitis: clinicopathological aspects of an emerging condition. Gut. 2012;61:1108–14.
18. Lamps LW. Infectious disorders of the upper gastrointestinal tract (excluding Helicobacter pylori). Diagn Histopathol. 2008;14:427–36.
19. Underwood JA, Williams JW, Keate RF. Clinical findings and risk factors for Candida esophagitis in outpatients. Dis Esophagus. 2003;16:66–9.
20. Canalejo F, Garcia Duran F, Cabello N, et al. Herpes esophagitis in healthy adults and adolescents: report of 3 cases and review of literature. Medicine (Baltimore). 2010;89:204–10.
21. Parfitt JR, Driman DK. Pathological effects of drugs on the gastrointestinal tract: a review. Hum Pathol. 2007;38:527–36.
22. Qiao WB, Zhao YH, Zhao YB, et al. Clinical and dosimetric factors of radiation-induced esophageal injury: radiation-induced esophageal toxicity. World J Gastroenterol. 2005;11:2626–9.
23. Galloro G, editor. Revisiting Barrett's esophagus. 1st ed. Vienna: Springer Verlag; 2019.
24. Shaheen NJ, Falk GW, Iyer PG. ACG clinical guideline: diagnosis and management of Barrett's esophagus. Am J Gastroenterol. 2016;111:30–50.
25. Hameeteman W, Tytgat GN, Houthoff HJ, et al. Barrett's esophagus: development of dysplasia and adenocarcinoma. Gastroenterology. 1989;96:1249–56.
26. Maione F, Chini A, Maione R, et al. Endoscopic diagnosis and management of Barrett's esophagus with low-grade dysplasia. Diagnostics (Basel). 2022;12(5):1295.
27. Levine DS, Blount PL, Rudolph RE. Safety of a systematic endoscopic biopsy protocol in patients with Barrett's esophagus. Am J Gastroenterol. 2000;95:1152–7.
28. Longcroft-Wheaton G, Brown J, Basford P. Duration of acetowhitening as a novel objective tool for diagnosing high risk neoplasia in Barrett's esophagus: a prospective cohort trial. Endoscopy. 2013;45:426–32.
29. Conio M, Blanchi S, Lapertosa G. Long-term endoscopic surveillance of patients with Barrett's esophagus. Incidence of dysplasia and adenocarcinoma: a prospective study. Am J Gastroenterol. 2003;98:1931–9.
30. Wani S, Falk GW, Post J. Risk factors for progression of low-grade dysplasia in patients with Barrett's esophagus. Gastroenterology. 2011;141:1179–86.
31. Weusten B, Bisschops R, Coron E. Endoscopic management of Barrett's esophagus: European Society of Gastrointestinal Endoscopy (ESGE) position statement. Endoscopy. 2017;49:191–8.
32. Qumseya B, Sultan S, Bain P. ASGE guideline on screening and surveillance of Barrett's esophagus. Gastrointest Endosc. 2019;90:335–9.
33. Gupta S, Li D, El Serag H. AGA clinical practice guidelines on management of gastric intestinal metaplasia. Gastroenterology. 2020;158:693–702.
34. Kew GS, Soh AYS, Lee YY. Multinational survey on the preferred approach to management of Barrett's esophagus in the Asia-Pacific region. World J Gastrointest Oncol. 2021;13:279–94.
35. Dam AN, Klapman J. A narrative review of Barrett's esophagus in 2020, molecular and clinical update. Ann Transl Med. 2020;8:1107.
36. Konda VJ, Gonzalez Haba Ruiz M, Koons A. Complete endoscopic mucosal resection is effective and durable treatment for Barrett's-associated neoplasia. Clin Gastroenterol Hepatol. 2014;12:2002–10.
37. Sami SS, Ravindran A, Kahn A. Timeline and location of recurrence following successful ablation in Barrett's oesophagus: an international multicentre study. Gut. 2019;68:1379–85.
38. Lal P, Thota PN. Cryotherapy in the management of premalignant and malignant conditions of the esophagus. World J Gastroenterol. 2018;24:4862–9.
39. Manner H, May A, Kouti I. Efficacy and safety of Hybrid-APC for the ablation of Barrett's esophagus. Surg Endosc. 2016;30:1364–70.

Open Access This chapter is licensed under the terms of the Creative Commons Attribution-NonCommercial 4.0 International License (http://creativecommons.org/licenses/by-nc/4.0/), which permits any noncommercial use, sharing, adaptation, distribution and reproduction in any medium or format, as long as you give appropriate credit to the original author(s) and the source, provide a link to the Creative Commons license and indicate if changes were made.

The images or other third party material in this chapter are included in the chapter's Creative Commons license, unless indicated otherwise in a credit line to the material. If material is not included in the chapter's Creative Commons license and your intended use is not permitted by statutory regulation or exceeds the permitted use, you will need to obtain permission directly from the copyright holder.

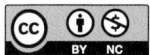

Medical Management

10

Marzio Frazzoni and Leonardo Frazzoni

10.1 Introduction

Gastroesophageal reflux disease (GERD) is defined as a condition which develops when the reflux of stomach contents causes troublesome symptoms and/or complications [1]. The typical reflux syndrome consists of heartburn with or without regurgitation, heartburn representing the most sensitive and specific GERD symptom. Atypical symptoms, including non-cardiac chest pain and extra-esophageal symptoms (cough, wheezing, hoarseness, throat clearing) are less common and specific, and often unrelated to reflux when thoroughly investigated. The prevalence of GERD is high, up to 20% in the Western world (20%) [2], so that it represents the most common disease encountered by gastroenterologists. Many factors contribute to GERD development, including weakness of the lower esophageal sphincter (LES), excess transient LES relaxations, displacement of the gastroesophageal junction above the diaphragm (sliding hiatal hernia), an enlarged unbuffered proximal gastric acid pocket, ineffective esophageal motility, impairment of esophageal volume and chemical clearance, and delayed gastric emptying [2]. Medical management includes lifestyle modifications and pharmacologic interventions [3].

10.2 Lifestyle Modifications

Weight loss for overweight and obese patients is strongly recommended [3], and even small amounts of weight loss can reduce GERD symptoms.

M. Frazzoni (✉)
Digestive Pathophysiology Unit, Baggiovara Hospital, Modena, Italy
e-mail: marziofrazzoni@gmail.com

L. Frazzoni
Gastroenterology and Digestive Endoscopy Unit, Bufalini Hospital, Cesena and Morgagni-Pierantoni Hospital, Forlì, Italy
e-mail: leonardo.frazzoni@gmail.com

© The Author(s) 2026
V. Landolfi, S. Tolone (eds.), *Functional Diseases of the Esophagus*, Updates in Surgery, https://doi.org/10.1007/978-3-031-90570-4_10

Other common recommendations include elevating the head of the bed, sleeping on the left side, tobacco and alcohol cessation, avoidance of late-night meals, snacks and alcoholic beverages, upright position during and after meals, avoidance of coffee, chocolate, carbonated drinks, and fatty, spicy and acidic foods [3]. Except for sleep with the head of the bed elevated and on the left side, evidence of efficacy for these recommendations is, however, limited [3].

10.3 Pharmacologic Intervention: Proton-Pump Inhibitors

Proton-pump inhibitors (PPIs) represent the mainstay of medical management for GERD [3]. Since plenty of data have demonstrated their outstanding efficacy in relieving heartburn, the cardinal GERD symptom, as well as in healing reflux esophagitis, they have become the most commonly prescribed medication for reflux symptoms.

PPIs owe their clinical efficacy to their ability to inhibit H^+K^+-adenosine triphosphatase in gastric parietal cells, resulting in suppression of gastric acid secretion: during PPI therapy, the majority of acid refluxes are transformed into weakly acidic refluxes, which are less harmful to the esophageal mucosa owing to the reduction of the proteolytic activity of pepsins when the environment becomes weakly acidic. Five PPIs are commercially available, and there are significant differences among them in terms of acid-suppressing activity and clinical efficacy, esomeprazole and pantoprazole being the most and the least efficient, respectively [4–9].

Of note, owing to their high efficacy in suppressing reflux symptoms PPIs have assumed an important role in the diagnostic work-up of GERD in clinical practice. Indeed, the diagnostic yield of upper GI endoscopy in GERD is low since erosive esophagitis and/or Barrett's esophagus can be detected in no more than 30% of cases; on the other hand, the diagnostic accuracy of pH-impedance monitoring is very high, particularly when novel pH-impedance metrics are assessed [10], but costs and complexity limit its use in daily clinical practice. Therefore, in the absence of alarm signs/symptoms (anemia, involuntary weight loss, GI bleeding, dysphagia, chest pain), a 4–8 week PPI trial resulting in symptomatic relief allows a presumptive GERD diagnosis in uninvestigated patients [3].

Over time, many PPI-responsive patients become PPI-dependent, requiring maintenance treatment with PPIs. In the SOPRAN study, at 12-year follow-up omeprazole with dose adjustments and open fundoplication were both effective and well tolerated, although the latter was associated with better control of overall GERD manifestations but persisting side effects [11]. In the LOTUS trial, the long-term efficacy of esomeprazole and laparoscopic fundoplication was compared in patients with erosive and non-erosive GERD [12]: in most cases, heartburn remission was maintained at 5-year follow-up either after surgery or with ongoing esomeprazole use, in a dose-escalating manner when required. Both these studies show persistent efficacy of maintenance PPI therapy over time, with dose adjustments when required. The safety of maintenance PPI therapy has been questioned, however, by several studies raising the suspicion of adverse effects related to prolonged

PPI use, including enteric infections, microscopic colitis, kidney disease, nutritional deficiencies, hypomagnesemia, gastric cancer, bone fractures, cardiovascular disease, dementia, and community-acquired pneumonia: however, the vast majority of such studies are flawed by major biases, and no cause-and-effect relationship has been definitely established [13]. Currently, long-term PPI therapy is strongly recommended for patients with GERD complications, including grade C/D reflux esophagitis (confluent/circumferential mucosal breaks), esophageal peptic strictures and Barrett's esophagus [3], and it is conditionally indicated in PPI-dependent mild (grade B) reflux esophagitis and non-erosive GERD as documented by pH/pH-impedance monitoring [14].

10.4 When Proton-Pump Inhibitors Fail

Despite the high efficacy of PPIs in suppressing reflux symptoms and healing esophageal mucosal breaks, heartburn and atypical reflux symptoms may persist in up to 20% and 50% of uninvestigated patients, respectively. In these cases, compliance must be checked since several patients do not take PPIs 30–60 min before the first meal of the day [15]. If compliance is adequate, twice-daily administration of the label dose may prove effective in significantly reducing acid reflux [15]. When symptoms persist despite twice-daily PPI therapy in uninvestigated patients, a diagnostic work-up preceded by two-week PPI withdrawal and consisting of off-therapy upper GI endoscopy and pH-impedance monitoring is warranted in order to distinguish reflux-related from reflux-unrelated (i.e., functional) symptoms, and diagnose or exclude GERD [16–18]. In PPI-refractory patients with documented GERD, on-PPI pH-impedance monitoring is required to distinguish reflux-related from functional symptoms [3, 15], amenable to either incremental antireflux management or neuromodulator treatment, respectively. The mechanism of PPI refractoriness can only be clarified by on-PPI pH-impedance monitoring: indeed, persistence of an excess weakly acidic reflux burden and severe impairment of esophageal chemical clearance unaffected by therapy represent the major causes of PPI refractoriness in patients with documented GERD [18–21], neither of the two detectable by on-PPI pH-only monitoring [22] even when combined with bile reflux monitoring [23].

In GERD patients with symptoms refractory to high-dose PPI therapy and due to ongoing reflux, laparoscopic fundoplication is a valuable management option, allowing persistent off-therapy heartburn suppression in up to 67–88% of cases at 1–3-year follow-up [18, 24, 25]. However, there are patients who are unfit for surgery or who fear the side effects and complications of laparoscopic fundoplication: for them, add-on and alternative medications to PPIs, as detailed below, are worthy of consideration.

H2-receptor antagonists (ranitidine, famotidine) may be added at bedtime for persisting nocturnal symptoms: efficacy is limited, however, since tachyphylaxis can arise after one month only [3, 15].

Prokinetics (metoclopramide, domperidone) must be avoided because of poor efficacy and dangerous side effects [3, 15].

Baclofen is a gamma-amino-butyric acid (GABA) receptor type B agonist which inhibits reflux events: when added to PPIs, it can improve reflux symptoms in cases with positive symptom association probability (SAP) as shown by on-PPI pH-impedance monitoring [26]. Unfortunately, side effects including dizziness, somnolence, and constipation limit its clinical use [3, 15].

A new formulation of a bile acid sequestrant (colesevelam) with a gastric retentive technology was investigated in a recent study as add-on therapy in patients with heartburn persistent on label-dose PPIs [27]: symptom relief was only modest, however, and the drug was not tested in patients with heartburn persisting on high-dose PPIs.

Alginate rapidly forms a physical barrier on top of the stomach contents in the form of a floating gel which localizes to the postprandial acid pocket and displaces it below the diaphragm to reduce postprandial acid reflux. When added to PPIs, alginate can improve heartburn control [28]. A formulation of hyaluronic acid and chondroitin-sulfate has recently been developed: it can be added to PPIs with improvement of persistent symptoms [29].

Recently, a new class of antisecretory agents named potassium-competitive acid blockers (P-CABs) has been developed [30], representing an alternative to PPIs. They reversibly bind to H+K+-ATPase to compete with potassium binding. Vonoprazan is the most widely investigated P-CAB [31]: it is acid-stable, thus eliminating the necessity for enteric coating and allowing for rapid onset of action. Vonoprazan rapidly achieves high and sustained (half-life 9 hours) concentrations in the parietal cell secretory canaliculi, so that maximal acid inhibition is achieved quickly after the first dose. Additionally, since it is not metabolized through the hepatic CYP2C19 or CYP3A4 enzymes, vonoprazan is much less prone to drug-drug interactions and to variability among individuals in the duration of action due to polymorphisms of these enzymes, as seen with PPIs. Vonoprazan was non-inferior to PPIs for GERD management in several studies. Of note, vonoprazan was more effective than lansoprazole in healing and maintenance of healing of severe (grade C/D) reflux esophagitis [32], while heartburn was relieved more promptly and more completely during the night-time with vonoprazan as compared with lansoprazole in patients with reflux esophagitis [33]. However, the remarkable acid suppression induced by vonoprazan needs careful monitoring for possible adverse events due to profound gastric acid suppression when long-term use is considered. Further, available data do not suggest any substantial advantage in heartburn relief of vonoprazan over the most potent PPI esomeprazole [34, 35]: thus, whenever vonoprazan is not available, shifting to esomeprazole 40 mg twice daily in patients unresponsive to the other PPIs may represent a valuable option.

In the current era of precision medicine, medical therapies should be tailored on the basis of individual rather than group analyses. On-PPI pH-impedance monitoring, besides establishing a direct link between reflux and on-therapy persistent symptoms, can also guide medical therapy [36], suggesting incremental acid suppression in cases of excess acid reflux or add-on antireflux medications in cases of excess weakly acidic reflux.

References

1. Vakil N, van Zanten SV, Kahrilas P, et al. The Montreal definition and classification of gastroesophageal reflux disease: a global evidence-based consensus. Am J Gastroenterol. 2006;101:1900–20.
2. Tack J, Pandolfino JE. Pathophysiology of gastroesophageal reflux disease. Gastroenterology. 2018;154:277–88.
3. Katz PO, Dunbar KB, Schnoll-Sussman FH, et al. ACG clinical guideline for the diagnosis and management of gastroesophageal reflux disease. Am J Gastroenterol. 2022;117:27–56.
4. Castell DO, Kahrilas PJ, Richter JE, et al. Esomeprazole (40 mg) compared with lansoprazole (30 mg) in the treatment of erosive esophagitis. Am J Gastroenterol. 2002;97:575–83.
5. Frazzoni M, De Micheli E, Grisendi A, Savarino V. Lansoprazole vs. omeprazole for gastro-oesophageal reflux disease: a pH-metric comparison. Aliment Pharmacol Ther. 2002;16:35–40.
6. Miner P, Katz PO, Chen Y, Sostek M. Gastric acid control with esomeprazole, lansoprazole, omeprazole, pantoprazole, and rabeprazole: a five-way crossover study. Am J Gastroenterol. 2003;98:2616–20.
7. Frazzoni M, De Micheli E, Grisendi A, Savarino V. Effective intra-oesophageal acid suppression in patients with gastro-oesophageal reflux disease: lansoprazole vs. pantoprazole. Aliment Pharmacol Ther. 2003;17:235–41.
8. Fennerty MB, Johanson JF, Hwang C, Sostek M. Efficacy of esomeprazole 40 mg vs. lansoprazole 30 mg for healing moderate to severe erosive oesophagitis. Aliment Pharmacol Ther. 2005;21:455–63.
9. Frazzoni M, Manno M, De Micheli E, Savarino V. Intra-oesophageal acid suppression in complicated gastro-oesophageal reflux disease: esomeprazole vs. lansoprazole. Dig Liver Dis. 2006;38:85–90.
10. Frazzoni M, Savarino E, De Bortoli N, et al. Analyses of the post-reflux swallow-induced peristaltic wave index and nocturnal baseline impedance parameters increase the diagnostic yield of impedance-pH monitoring of patients with reflux disease. Clin Gastroenterol Hepatol. 2016;14:40–6.
11. Lundell L, Miettinen P, Myrvold HE, et al. Comparison of outcomes twelve years after antireflux surgery or omeprazole maintenance therapy for reflux esophagitis. Clin Gastroenterol Hepatol. 2009;7:1292–8.
12. Galmiche JP, Hatlebakk J, Attwood S, et al. Laparoscopic antireflux surgery vs esomeprazole treatment for chronic GERD – the LOTUS randomized clinical trial. JAMA. 2011;305:1969–77.
13. Savarino V, Marabotto E, Furnari M, et al. Latest insights into the hot question of proton pump inhibitor safety – a narrative review. Dig Liver Dis. 2020;52:842–52.
14. Targownik LE, Fisher DA, Saini SD. AGA clinical practice update on de-prescribing of proton pump inhibitors: expert review. Gastroenterology. 2022;162:1334–42.
15. Zerbib F, Bredenoord AJ, Fass R, et al. ESNM/ANMS consensus paper: diagnosis and management of refractory gastro-esophageal reflux disease. Neurogastroenterol Motil. 2021;33:e14075.
16. Trudgill NJ, Sifrim D, Sweis R, et al. British Society of Gastroenterology guidelines for oesophageal manometry and oesophageal reflux monitoring. Gut. 2019;68:1731–50.
17. Frazzoni L, Frazzoni M, De Bortoli N, et al. Application of Lyon consensus criteria for GORD diagnosis: evaluation of conventional and new impedance-pH parameters. Gut. 2022;71:1062–7.
18. Frazzoni M, Frazzoni L, Ribolsi M, et al. Applying Lyon consensus criteria in the work-up of patients with proton pump inhibitory-refractory heartburn. Aliment Pharmacol Ther. 2022;55:1423–30.
19. Frazzoni M, Conigliaro R, Melotti G. Weakly acidic refluxes have a major role in the pathogenesis of proton pump inhibitor-resistant reflux oesophagitis. Aliment Pharmacol Ther. 2011;33:601–6.

20. Frazzoni M, Bertani H, Manta R, et al. Impairment of chemical clearance is relevant to the pathogenesis of refractory reflux oesophagitis. Dig Liver Dis. 2014;46:596–602.
21. Frazzoni M, Frazzoni L, Tolone S, et al. Lack of improvement of impaired chemical clearance characterizes PPI-refractory reflux-related heartburn. Am J Gastroenterol. 2018;113:670–6.
22. Charbel S, Khandwala F, Vaezi MF. The role of esophageal pH monitoring in symptomatic patients on PPI therapy. Am J Gastroenterol. 2005;100:283–9.
23. Gasiorowska A, Navarro-Rodriguez T, Wendel C, et al. Comparison of the degree of duodenogastroesophageal reflux and acid reflux between patients who failed to respond and those who were successfully treated with a proton pump inhibitor once daily. Am J Gastroenterol. 2009;104:2005–13.
24. Frazzoni M, Piccoli M, Conigliaro R, et al. Refractory gastroesophageal reflux disease as diagnosed by impedance-pH monitoring can be cured by laparoscopic fundoplication. Surg Endosc. 2013;27:2940–6.
25. Spechler SJ, Hunter JG, Jones KM, et al. Randomized trial of medical versus surgical treatment for refractory heartburn. N Engl J Med. 2019;381:1513–23.
26. Pauwels A, Raymenants K, Geeraerts A, et al. Clinical trial: a controlled trial of baclofen add-on therapy in PPI-refractory gastro-esophageal reflux symptoms. Aliment Pharmacol Ther. 2022;56:231–9.
27. Vaezi MF, Fass R, Vakil N, et al. IW-3718 reduces heartburn severity in patients with refractory gastroesophageal reflux disease in a randomized trial. Gastroenterology. 2020;158:2093–103.
28. Reimer C, Lødrup AB, Smith G, et al. Randomised clinical trial: alginate (Gaviscon advance) vs. placebo as add-on therapy in reflux patients with inadequate response to a once daily proton pump inhibitor. Aliment Pharmacol Ther. 2016;43:899–909.
29. Savarino V, Pace F, Scarpignato C, et al. Randomised clinical trial: mucosal protection combined with acid suppression in the treatment of non-erosive reflux disease-efficacy of Esoxx, a hyaluronic acid-chondroitin sulphate based bioadhesive formulation. Aliment Pharmacol Ther. 2017;45:631–42.
30. Leowattana W, Leowattana T. Potassium-competitive acid blockers and gastroesophageal reflux disease. World J Gastroenterol. 2022;28:3608–19.
31. Savarino V, Antonioli L, Fornai M, et al. An update of pharmacology, efficacy, and safety of vonoprazan in acid-related disorders. Expert Rev Gastroenterol Hepatol. 2022;16:401–10.
32. Laine L, DeVault K, Katz P, et al. Vonoprazan versus lansoprazole for healing and maintenance of healing of erosive esophagitis: a randomized trial. Gastroenterology. 2023;164:61–71.
33. Oshima T, Arai E, Taki M, et al. Randomised clinical trial: vonoprazan vs lansoprazole for the initial relief of heartburn in patients with erosive oesophagitis. Aliment Pharmacol Ther. 2019;49:140–6.
34. Tack J, Vladimirov B, Horny I, et al. Randomized clinical trial: a double-blind, proof-of-concept, phase 2 study evaluating the efficacy and safety of vonoprazan 20 or 40 mg versus esomeprazole 40 mg in patients with symptomatic gastro-esophageal reflux disease and partial response to a healing dose of a proton-pump inhibitor. Neurogastroenterol Motil. 2023;35:e14468.
35. Zhuang Q, Chen S, Zhou X, et al. Comparative efficacy of P-CAB vs proton pump inhibitors for grade C/D esophagitis: a systematic review and network meta-analysis. Am J Gastroenterol. 2024;119:803–13.
36. Frazzoni M, Frazzoni L, Ribolsi M, et al. On-therapy impedance-pH monitoring can efficiently characterize PPI-refractory GERD and support treatment escalation. Neurogastroenterol Motil. 2023;35:e14547.

Open Access This chapter is licensed under the terms of the Creative Commons Attribution-NonCommercial 4.0 International License (http://creativecommons.org/licenses/by-nc/4.0/), which permits any noncommercial use, sharing, adaptation, distribution and reproduction in any medium or format, as long as you give appropriate credit to the original author(s) and the source, provide a link to the Creative Commons license and indicate if changes were made.

The images or other third party material in this chapter are included in the chapter's Creative Commons license, unless indicated otherwise in a credit line to the material. If material is not included in the chapter's Creative Commons license and your intended use is not permitted by statutory regulation or exceeds the permitted use, you will need to obtain permission directly from the copyright holder.

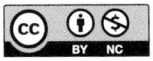

Diet

11

Antonella Santonicola, Ida de Micco, Luigi Schiavo, and Paola Iovino

11.1 Introduction

Esophageal disorders, including gastroesophageal reflux disease (GERD), are influenced by multiple factors, with dietary habits being among the major contributors to the onset and exacerbation of symptoms. In fact, dietary habits can significantly affect esophageal function and motility through several mechanisms, which include altering the lower esophageal sphincter (LES) pressure, modifying gastric acid secretion, and affecting esophageal peristalsis.

11.2 The Effect of Dietary Components on Lower Esophageal Sphincter Pressure

LES is a tonically contracted band of muscle that relaxes transiently to allow the passage of food and liquids into the stomach and contracts to prevent reflux of gastric contents. Both intrinsic and extrinsic factors, including neural, hormonal, and dietary components influence LES pressure. LES basal tone is maintained by the myogenic properties of the smooth muscle and modulated by neural inputs, primarily via the vagus nerve. Hormones such as gastrin, motilin, and ghrelin can increase LES pressure, whereas hormones like cholecystokinin and secretin tend to decrease it [1]. Dietary components and eating habits play a significant role in modulating LES pressure, with some foods playing a major role in the onset of some symptoms [2].

A. Santonicola · I. de Micco · L. Schiavo · P. Iovino (✉)
Department of Medicine, Surgery, and Dentistry, Scuola Medica Salernitana, University of Salerno, Baronissi, Italy
e-mail: asantonicola@unisa.it; idademicco@gmail.com; lschiavo@unisa.it; piovino@unisa.it

- **High-fat foods**. High-fat food intake reduces LES pressure and increases esophageal exposure to gastric fluids. A systematic review investigating the relationship between GERD occurrence and different foods and dietary patterns found a significant relationship between adherence to high-fat diets and increased risk of GERD [3]. Consumption of large, high-fat meals was associated with increased acid exposure time in patients compared to low-fat meals and accelerated the development of GERD by reducing LES pressure. In fact, high-fat meals delay gastric emptying and may cause prolonged gastric distension, which can reduce LES tone, as demonstrated in a study by Penagini et al. [4]. This is also due to the increased production of bile acids and pepsin in response to fatty foods. These substances are particularly damaging to the esophageal mucosa and can lead to inflammation and esophagitis, as shown by Sifrim et al. [5]. Dietary fats can influence the release of hormones that regulate LES pressure and gastric motility. For example, cholecystokinin (CCK) is released in response to fatty meals and is known to decrease LES pressure. This hormonal modulation adds another layer of complexity to how high-fat diets promote reflux [6].
- **Fibers**. Dietary fiber, particularly soluble fiber, forms a gelatinous substance when it dissolves in water, increasing gastric content viscosity and slowing down the gastric emptying process. Moreover, the bulk formation leads to greater gastric distension, which can activate gastric stretch receptors, signaling the need to slow gastric emptying to manage the increased volume effectively [7]. Fibers also influence the contractions of the stomach muscles, increasing the frequency and strength of contractions that help in mixing the food but slow down its progression to the pylorus. This modulation ensures a more gradual and consistent emptying process, preventing large volumes of food from entering the small intestine too quickly, which can engulf the digestive processes. High-fiber foods seem to impact the acidity of the stomach contents, as fibers tend to buffer stomach acids, contributing to maintaining an optimal pH for the activity of digestive enzymes like pepsin. This buffering effect, coupled with slower gastric emptying, ensures that the chyme is adequately mixed with digestive enzymes and is thoroughly digested before it moves to the small intestine, and is crucial for preventing undigested food particles from irritating the esophagus and LES [8]. Lastly, fibers stimulate the release of gastrin, CCK, and peptide YY (PYY), which play crucial roles in regulating gastric emptying. For example, CCK slows gastric emptying by relaxing the proximal stomach and contracting the pyloric sphincter, thereby prolonging the retention time of food in the stomach, which helps in maintaining a slower and more controlled release of stomach contents into the small intestine. The extended digestion time also promotes a feeling of satiety, which can help in weight management. Since obesity is a risk factor for GERD, the satiety-inducing properties of fiber can indirectly contribute to improved esophageal health by aiding in weight control.
- **Chocolate and peppermint**. Both chocolate and peppermint have been shown to reduce LES pressure, possibly due to their methylxanthine content. Methylaxanthine, which inhibits the activity of phosphodiesterases and acts as non-selective antagonist of adenosine receptors seems effective at promoting

smooth muscle relaxation, including LES [9]. Shay et al. found that chocolate consumption significantly decreased LES pressure and increased acid exposure in the esophagus [10].
- **Caffeine**. Caffeinated beverages such as coffee and tea can increase gastric acid secretion and decrease LES pressure. Caffeine, which is a major methylxanthine in coffee and tea, inhibits phosphodiesterases and acts as a non-selective antagonist of adenosine receptors, therefore decreasing intracellular calcium concentrations. Caffeine may also exert direct effects on smooth muscle cells by interfering with calcium release from the sarcoplasmic reticulum and inhibiting calcium influx through calcium channels, contributing to the relaxation of LES smooth muscle and the overall reduction in LES pressure [11]. Moreover, Wendl et al. reported that decaffeinated coffee had less of an impact on LES pressure compared to regular coffee, suggesting caffeine as a key factor [12].
- **Alcohol**. Alcohol consumption is well known to influence the function of LES, often leading to its relaxation and an increased risk of gastroesophageal reflux. Ethanol increases the production and release of nitric oxide from the enteric nervous system which activates guanylate cyclase in smooth muscle cells, leading to an increase in cyclic guanosine monophosphate (cGMP) [9]. Elevated cGMP levels activate protein kinase G (PKG), which subsequently reduces intracellular calcium levels and promotes smooth muscle relaxation [9]. Ethanol has been shown to interfere directly with calcium in the LES smooth muscle cells, reducing calcium influx through voltage-dependent calcium channels and inhibiting calcium release from the sarcoplasmic reticulum [13]. This reduction in intracellular calcium levels diminishes the contractile force of the smooth muscle, leading to LES relaxation [13]. Moreover, ethanol consumption can enhance the release of inhibitory neurotransmitters, such as vasoactive intestinal peptide (VIP), which can increase the release of CCK, which binds to receptors on LES smooth muscle cells and reduces LES pressure. Alcohol may also exacerbate inflammation and oxidative stress within the gastrointestinal tract, promoting the production of inflammatory cytokines and reactive oxygen species (ROS), which can impair the function of the smooth muscle cells and the enteric nervous system, further promoting LES dysfunction [11]. These combined effects result in a significant reduction in LES pressure and explain why alcohol consumption is a common risk factor for GERD and related symptoms.

11.3 The Role of Dietary Interventions in Esophageal Health

According to international guidelines, one of the most crucial treatments for patients suffering from GERD is dietary modification. Several intervention studies utilizing low-carb, high-fat, and low-FODMAP diets have been conducted to assess the efficacy of various nutritional interventions in GERD patients. However, to date, there is insufficient data to support the effectiveness of these dietary approaches, since most of the recommendations are based on uncontrolled studies [14]. Figure 11.1 shows the possible effect of the different dietary interventions on esophageal health.

Fig. 11.1 Possible effect of the different dietary interventions on esophageal health

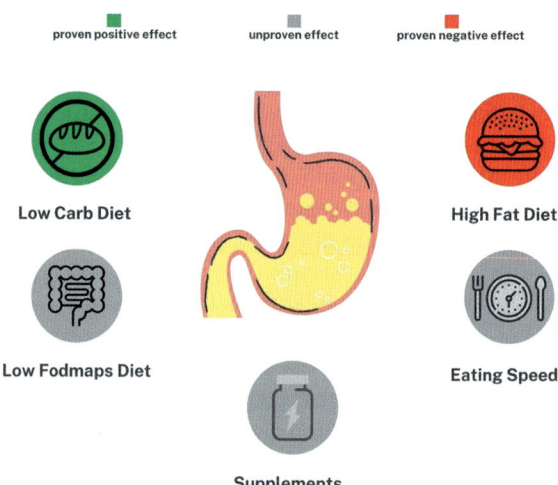

11.3.1 Low-Carbohydrate Diet

A few studies showed improved GERD symptoms after low-carbohydrate diets [15–17]. A 2006 study on eight GERD patients with obesity (BMI >30 kg/m^2) conducted by Austin et al. [15] showed that a low-carbohydrate diet (less than 20 g/day) for 3–6 days significantly reduced GERD symptoms, as evaluated by the GERD Symptom Assessment Scale-Distress Subscale (GSAS-ds). The authors also demonstrated that after a low-carbohydrate diet, there was an improvement in the pH monitoring parameters, with a significant reduction in the acid exposure time (AET) (5.1 ± 1.3% before diet vs. 2.5 ± 0.6% after diet; p = 0.022). The randomized controlled trial cross-over study by Wu et al. [16] confirmed these results; the authors, in fact, reported a worsening in reflux symptoms after a high-carbohydrate diet in GERD patients. Moreover, pH monitoring parameters such as DeMeester score, total reflux time, and number of reflux periods were significantly higher after the high-carbohydrate diet (p < 0.05). Further evidence of a reduction in GERD symptoms after a low-carbohydrate diet comes from the randomized controlled dietary intervention trial by Gu et al. [17], showing that a change in dietary carbohydrate intake aimed at significantly reducing the intake of simple sugars improved pH monitoring results and symptoms of GERD. A recent meta-analysis [14] confirmed the significant decrease in esophageal acid exposure after low-carbohydrate diets compared to high-carbohydrate diets. However, the underlying mechanisms have not been completely clarified yet. Among the proposed mechanisms, there is the effect on gastric distension. In fact, a high-carbohydrate meal could occupy a larger gastric volume; moreover, some carbohydrates, such as lactose and FODMAP could increase the number of transient lower esophageal relaxations (TLESRs) [18] favouring reflux. The effect of low-carbohydrate diets on GERD does not seem to be linked to weight loss, as the beneficial effects of this diet are revealed in the short term, in patients without significant weight loss.

11.3.2 High-Fat Diet

In clinical practice, physicians often suggest to GERD patients to avoid high-fat foods, since they could delay gastric emptying and increase reflux symptoms. However, the effects of a high-fat diet on GERD are still conflicting [14]. In a 1998 study, Penagini et al. [19] demonstrated no significant difference in esophageal acid exposure and the number of reflux episodes in GERD patients after a high-fat meal (44 g fat) compared to a balanced meal (20 g fat). Their results were also confirmed by another Italian study on 13 healthy subjects who underwent 6-h esophageal pH monitoring after three meals of the same volume and osmolarity but different fat content and caloric load: a) high fat (58% fat) 2.8 MJ; b) balanced (23% fat) 2.8 MJ; and c) balanced low calorie (25% fat) 1.6 MJ. The authors demonstrated that the effect on GERD was related to the caloric load of meals rather than their fat content [20]. In contrast, Fan et al. [21], in their study on 27 patients with GERD, found a significantly higher percentage of esophageal acid exposure at 4 hours (median 5, 2% vs. 4%) when comparing a high-fat meal to a standard meal.

11.3.3 Low-FODMAP Diet

A diet low in fermentable oligosaccharides, disaccharides, monosaccharides, and polyols (FODMAPs) reduces the ingestion of poorly absorbed short-chain carbohydrates, such as lactose or fructooligosaccharides. Patients with irritable bowel syndrome (IBS) usually improve their gastrointestinal symptoms during this type of diet, probably thanks to the reduction of colonic microbial fermentation [22]. A multicenter, randomized, open-label study by Riviere et al. [23] compared the effect on reflux of a 4-week low-FODMAP diet vs. usual dietary advice such as low-fat diet and postural measures in 31 patients with symptomatic proton-pump inhibitor (PPI) refractory GERD. The authors concluded that the low-FODMAP diet did not seem more effective than usual dietary advice in patients with PPI-refractory GERD symptoms and suggested recommending a low-FODMAP diet only in patients with concomitant IBS. Another recent, small study on eight patients evaluated the effect of the low-FODMAP diet in patients with overlapping GERD-IBS, showing that postprandial regurgitation (2.9±1.2 vs. 0.4±0.2), bloating (7.0±0.4 vs. 3.1±0.9), satiety (7.7±0.4 vs. 3.5±0.9), and belching (3.8±1.2 vs. 1.1±0.6) symptom scores were significantly greater after a high-FODMAP diet ($p < 0.05$). Furthermore, a high-FODMAP diet was associated with a higher frequency of TLESRs [24].

11.3.4 Other Dietary Interventions

11.3.4.1 Eating Speed
Physicians often suggest to GERD patients to chew food thoroughly and eat slowly. Eating speed was evaluated in several studies. Riviere et al. [23] compared fast (within 5 min) and slow (within 30 min) eating in 46 patients with GERD; they did

not find any statistically significant differences in total reflux events within 3 h of ingestion. Another study by Bor et al. [25] confirmed that the total reflux events, the total reflux time, and reflux symptoms within 3 h were similar in fast or slow-eating GERD patients.

11.3.4.2 Dietary Supplements

Bor et al. compared dietary supplements (melatonin, vitamins, and amino acids) with a daily regimen of 20 mg omeprazole; the results showed a significant improvement in GERD symptoms in the dietary supplement group (100% vs. 65.7% in the omeprazole group, p = 0.001). However, the efficacy of the treatment was evaluated considering the time to achieve the first 24 hours without GERD symptoms; moreover, 90% of patients reported somnolence in the dietary supplement group [26].

Another study demonstrated that a 10-day diet with soluble fibers had a beneficial effect on non-erosive reflux disease (NERD), achieving a 7-day heartburn-free period in 60% of patients and an improvement in their GERD-Q scores. However, no changes in the pH monitoring parameters were found [27].

11.4 Conclusion

Although clinicians generally suggest dietary interventions as a first step of therapy for GERD patients, current evidence about this topic is still scanty. A meta-analysis confirmed the positive effect of low-carbohydrate diets on GERD but did not show any improvement with other dietary regimens. However, most intervention studies contained small numbers of patients with a high heterogeneity. Furthermore, the follow-up period is short, and GERD diagnosis often relies only on patients' reported symptoms. Therefore, a tailored approach is needed to achieve the goals of these dietary interventions for each patient. Unnecessary dietary restrictions should be avoided, as the effect of most dietary interventions could not be confirmed by current evidence and may result in a reduced quality of life and inadequate nutritional intake, especially in malnourished patients.

References

1. Kahrilas PJ, Pandolfino JE. Gastroesophageal reflux disease and its complications. In: Feldman M, Friedman LS, Brandt LJ, editors. Sleisenger and Fordtran's gastrointestinal and liver disease. 10th ed. Philadelphia: Saunders; 2016. p. 905–36.
2. Yadlapati R, Pandolfino JE. Esophageal motility disorders: advances in diagnosis and treatment. Gastroenterology. 2018;154(7):1906–19.
3. Heidarzadeh-Esfahani N, Soleimani D, Hajiahmadi S, et al. Dietary intake in relation to the risk of reflux disease: a systematic review. Prev Nutr Food Sci. 2021;26(4):367–79.
4. Penagini R, Mangano M, Amato M, et al. Mechanisms of gastro-oesophageal reflux in patients with systemic sclerosis. Gut. 2013;62(3):323–9.

5. Sifrim D, Castell D, Dent J, Kahrilas PJ. Gastroesophageal reflux monitoring: review and consensus report on detection and definitions of acid, non-acid, and gas reflux. Gut. 2004;53(7):1024–31.
6. Goyal RK, Chaudhury A. Physiology of normal esophageal motility. J Clin Gastroenterol. 2008;42(5):610–9.
7. Zhang Y, Chen H, Lu M, et al. Dietary fiber intake reduces risk for gastroesophageal reflux disease: a meta-analysis. Clin Gastroenterol Hepatol. 2018;16(11):1626–35.
8. Feinle C, O'Donovan D, Doran S, et al. Effects of fat digestion on appetite, APD motility, and gut hormones in response to duodenal fat infusion in humans. Am J Physiol Gastrointest Liver Physiol. 2003;284(5):G798–807.
9. Konturek PC, Konturek SJ, Brzozowski T, et al. Role of nitric oxide in gastroprotection and gastric adaptation to injury: interaction with prostaglandins. J Physiol Pharmacol. 2003;54(1):1–17.
10. Shay H, Goyal RK, Pal J, Cohen S. Mechanism of action of chocolate on lower esophageal sphincter. Am J Clin Nutr. 2005;41(6):1172–5.
11. Feldman M, Schiller LR. Disorders of gastrointestinal motility associated with diabetes mellitus. Ann Intern Med. 1983;98(3):378–84.
12. Wendl B, Pfeiffer A, Pehl C, et al. Effect of decaffeination of coffee or tea on gastro-oesophageal reflux. Aliment Pharmacol Ther. 2017;46(3):283–7.
13. Gillis RA, Quest JA, Pagani FD, Norman WP. Control centers in the central nervous system for regulating gastrointestinal motility. In: Johnson LR, editor. Physiology of the gastrointestinal tract. 3rd ed. New York: Raven Press; 1994. p. 621–83.
14. Lakananurak N, Pitisuttithum P, Susantitaphong P, et al. The efficacy of dietary interventions in patients with gastroesophageal reflux disease: a systematic review and meta-analysis of intervention studies. Nutrients. 2024;16(3):464.
15. Austin GL, Thiny MT, Westman EC, et al. A very low-carbohydrate diet improves gastro-esophageal reflux and its symptoms. Dig Dis Sci. 2006;51(8):1307–12.
16. Wu KL, Kuo CM, Yao CC, et al. The effect of dietary carbohydrate on gastroesophageal reflux disease. J Formos Med Assoc. 2018;117(11):973–8.
17. Gu C, Olszewski T, King KL, et al. The effects of modifying amount and type of dietary carbohydrate on esophageal acid exposure time and esophageal reflux symptoms: a randomized controlled trial. Am J Gastroenterol. 2022;117(10):1655–67.
18. Bove M, Lundell L, Ny L, et al. Effects of dietary nitrate on oesophageal motor function and gastro-oesophageal acid exposure in healthy volunteers and reflux patients. Digestion. 2003;68:49–56.
19. Penagini R, Mangano M, Bianchi PA. Effect of increasing the fat content but not the energy load of a meal on gastro-oesophageal reflux and lower oesophageal sphincter motor function. Gut. 1998;42(3):330–3.
20. Colombo P, Mangano M, Bianchi PA, Penagini R. Effect of calories and fat on postprandial gastro-oesophageal reflux. Scand J Gastroenterol. 2002;37(1):3–5.
21. Fan WJ, Hou YT, Sun XH, et al. Effect of high-fat, standard, and functional food meals on esophageal and gastric pH in patients with gastroesophageal reflux disease and healthy subjects. J Dig Dis. 2018;19(11):664–73.
22. Sloan TJ, Jalanka J, Major GAD, et al. A low FODMAP diet is associated with changes in the microbiota and reduction in breath hydrogen but not colonic volume in healthy subjects. PLoS One. 2018;13(7):e0201410.
23. Rivière P, Vauquelin B, Rolland E, et al. Low FODMAPs diet or usual dietary advice for the treatment of refractory gastroesophageal reflux disease: an open-labeled randomized trial. Neurogastroenterol Motil. 2021;33(9):e14181.
24. Plaidum S, Patcharatrakul T, Promjampa W, Gonlachanvit S. The effect of fermentable, oligosaccharides, disaccharides, monosaccharides, and polyols (FODMAP) meals on transient lower esophageal relaxations (TLESR) in gastroesophageal reflux disease (GERD) patients with overlapping irritable bowel syndrome (IBS). Nutrients. 2022;14(9):1755.

25. Bor S, Bayrakci B, Erdogan A, et al. The influence of the speed of food intake on multichannel impedance in patients with gastro-oesophageal reflux disease. United Eur Gastroenterol J. 2013;1(4):346–50.
26. Bor S, Erdogan A, Bayrakci B, et al. The impact of the speed of food intake on gastroesophageal reflux events in obese female patients. Dis Esophagus. 2017;30(1):1–6.
27. Morozov S, Isakov V, Konovalova M. Fiber-enriched diet helps to control symptoms and improves esophageal motility in patients with non-erosive gastroesophageal reflux disease. World J Gastroenterol. 2018;24(20):2291–9.

Open Access This chapter is licensed under the terms of the Creative Commons Attribution-NonCommercial 4.0 International License (http://creativecommons.org/licenses/by-nc/4.0/), which permits any noncommercial use, sharing, adaptation, distribution and reproduction in any medium or format, as long as you give appropriate credit to the original author(s) and the source, provide a link to the Creative Commons license and indicate if changes were made.

The images or other third party material in this chapter are included in the chapter's Creative Commons license, unless indicated otherwise in a credit line to the material. If material is not included in the chapter's Creative Commons license and your intended use is not permitted by statutory regulation or exceeds the permitted use, you will need to obtain permission directly from the copyright holder.

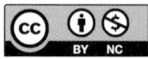

Rehabilitation

12

Adriana Maria Landolfi

12.1 Introduction

Esophageal disorders have a significant impact on the patient's quality of life. Pharmacological therapies and surgery resolve the symptoms in most cases, but for some years, physiotherapy has been considered an adjunct in managing these conditions, with exciting results especially in the long term. Physiotherapy acts on gastroesophageal disorders reflexively, working with diaphragmatic breathing training and postural re-education. The diaphragm is a skeletal muscle that divides the thoracic cavity from the abdominal cavity. It is dome-shaped and has contacts with the esophagus, stomach, ribs (from the 7th to the 12th), pericardium, and lumbar area through its diaphragmatic pillars. Given its size, it is divided into:

- Crural diaphragm (CD), which has a minor respiratory role because it does not significantly change the dimensions of the rib cage but is heavily involved in gastroesophageal functions;
- Costal diaphragm, which has the role of expanding the lower rib cage [1, 2].

Some scientific studies have shown that 85% of the contractility of the esophagogastric junction is attributable to the diaphragm [3]. Since the diaphragm is a skeletal muscle, and therefore partially voluntary, its dysfunctions can be improved with various respiratory rehabilitation techniques. Objective evaluations such as high-resolution manometry (HRM) have been performed before and after respiratory rehabilitation in patients with hypotensive lower esophageal sphincter (LES). Manometric evaluation showed an increase in the tone of the LES after diaphragmatic respiratory rehabilitation both at rest and during swallowing. This evaluation

A. M. Landolfi (✉)
Istituto Scientifico Euromedica, Milan, Italy
e-mail: adrianalandolfi@hotmail.it

was also performed in patients with ineffective esophageal motility (IEM), showing surprising results after rehabilitation [4].

HRM helps evaluate the integrity of the antireflux barrier by considering parameters such as basal LES tone, presence of LES-CD separation, and esophageal contractile vigor. Considering that 85% of the esophagogastric junction contractility is attributable to the diaphragm, the question to ask is how this occurs. Among the numerous scientific studies, some have focused on the effect of increased intra-abdominal pressure (IAP) on the esophagogastric junction. The increase in IAP was simulated in three different ways:

1. Using a pneumatic pressure cuff inflated to 50 and 100 mmHg;
2. Using the Valsalva maneuver sustained for at least 20 seconds;
3. Using the Lasegue test (also known as straight leg raise test), which involves raising the straight leg from a supine position. This position was maintained for at least 20 seconds.

The diaphragm muscle tone was evaluated using electromyography during abdominal compression, adding important information about diaphragm function. The result was that the tonic activity of the diaphragm increased during abdominal pressure loading, and was proportional to the amount of the load. Therefore, the authors hypothesized a "stretch reflex" from the diaphragmatic muscle spindles contributing to diaphragmatic tone, even if they could not exclude other mechanisms such as a vagal reflex. A common result in all studies was an increased LES pressure in response to increased IAP in asymptomatic volunteers and patients with normal LES pressure and length. However, in patients with symptomatic gastroesophageal reflux disease (GERD), the increase in LES pressure during rises in IAP was lower and not directly proportional to the amount of the load [5].

Posture is also important because a spinal problem, such as dorsal hyperkyphosis or lumbar hyperlordosis, can alter the diaphragm functionality, which consequently affects the integrity of the antireflux barrier.

The rehabilitation program consists of a multidisciplinary approach that includes:

- Postural examination;
- Specific diaphragmatic breathing exercises;
- Dietary re-education;
- Psychological support.

12.2 Postural Examination

Postural examination consists of an analysis of body movements aimed at evaluating the patient's posture. It is carried out with or without the use of specific instruments to identify any musculoskeletal alterations. The evaluation is performed in three spatial planes:

- In the frontal plane, anteriorly, the inclination and rotation of the head, the position of the shoulders and clavicles, the position of the knees (possible varus or valgus), and the foot support are evaluated; in the frontal plane, posteriorly, the scapulae, the axis of the humeri, the width of the waist triangles, the rotation of the pelvis, the axis of the femurs, and the foot support are evaluated;
- In the sagittal plane, any alterations in the physiological curves of the spine are evaluated;
- In the horizontal plane, the rotations of the shoulder and pelvic girdles are evaluated.

Based on the detected postural dysfunctions, a tailored rehabilitation program is created for each patient, which will allow the body to be realigned and rebalanced in bilateral harmony. This program includes stretching exercises for the muscle chains and strengthening exercises for the dorsal, abdominal, and antigravity muscles. Additionally, the physiotherapist's task is to correct the patients' posture by making them aware of their alterations so they can use correct posture during daily activities.

12.3 Specific Breathing Exercises

Because the diaphragm plays an extremely important role in the antireflux barrier, it is essential to improve its functionality. As is known, there are three types of breathing: thoracic, diaphragmatic, and mixed.

The type of breathing to be used to improve the functionality and elasticity of the diaphragm is diaphragmatic breathing, where during inhalation the diaphragm contracts and lowers to allow the lungs to fill with air while the belly swells; conversely, during exhalation, it relaxes and rises, allowing partial emptying of the lungs.

For optimal activation of the diaphragm, it is important that the ideal line of the chest is parallel to that of the pelvis, assuming a caudal position of the chest (Fig. 12.1). To achieve this position, the guidance of a physiotherapist during the execution of various exercises is required. To achieve long-term results, it is also important to perform at least 30 minutes of exercises per day.

In a systematic review, Lucie Zdrhova and colleagues reported on 11 clinical trials investigating the effects of respiratory rehabilitation in patients with non-erosive gastroesophageal reflux disease (NERD) [4]. One of these studies, a randomized controlled trial by Eherer et al., assessed quality of life, pHmetry, and on-demand use of proton-pump inhibitors (PPIs) before and after the end of a 4-week rehabilitation program consisting of diaphragmatic breathing exercises performed for 30 minutes a day; moreover, participants were instructed to continue the breathing exercises after the end of the study period, and their quality of life and PPI use were reassessed at 9 months. In all patients who underwent rehabilitation, there was a significant reduction in esophageal acid exposure time compared to the control group. Additionally, the patients who continued to do 30 minutes of exercises a day for

Fig. 12.1 Above: wrong position; below: caudal position of the chest

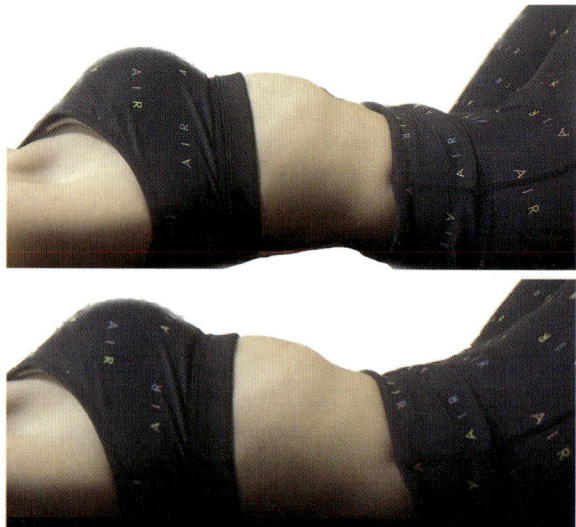

9 months showed a one-third reduction in the use of PPIs compared to baseline, as well as an improvement in quality of life [4].

Below are some exercises to be adopted within a respiratory rehabilitation program:

Exercise 1—Proprioception

Starting from a supine position with bent legs, the patient should perform five thoracic breaths and five diaphragmatic breaths to better understand the type of breathing to be performed. Thoracic breathing involves inhaling through the nose, which causes the chest to expand and the shoulders to lift, and ends with exhaling through the mouth, returning to the initial position. Diaphragmatic breathing involves inhaling through the nose, during which the belly inflates, and slowly exhaling, deflating it. To better perceive the correct movement, the patient can be instructed to place their hands on their belly (Fig. 12.2).

Exercise 2—Deep Exhalation

Starting from a supine position with bent legs, the patient should inhale through the nose, inflating the belly, and exhale through the mouth, blowing out for at least 20 seconds without forcing. It is difficult for the patient to perform the exercise correctly immediately, so the exhalation times should be gradually extended by performing the exercise regularly [6].

Exercise 3—Reverse Diaphragmatic Exhalation

Starting from a supine position with bent legs, the patient should inhale through the nose, inflating the belly, and exhale through the mouth, blowing out for 15–20 seconds while keeping the belly inflated. During the exercise, the chest should slowly lower. This exercise promotes stretching of the intercostal muscles.

Fig. 12.2 Proprioception exercise

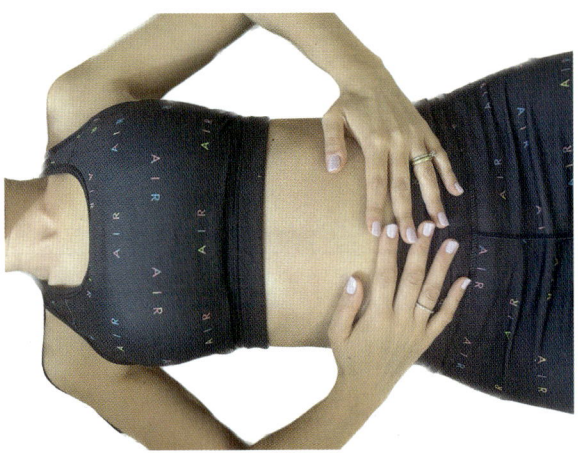

Exercise 4—Massage Therapy

Massage therapy performed by the physiotherapist at the abdominal and subcostal level helps reduce abdominal tensions and contractions that prevent the correct execution of the exercises. It is therefore extremely important to use decontracting massage techniques to promote the greatest possible stretching of the muscles, allowing for deeper and more correct breathing. Subsequently, the patient will be taught self-massage to continue the exercise at home.

12.4   Dietary Re-education

Nutrition is one of the first points of focus in the case of esophageal diseases. As mentioned in the previous chapter, it is essential that the patient follows the dietary guidelines and balanced diet indicated by the specialist based on the esophageal pathology and the reported symptoms.

12.5   Psychological Support

Some esophageal diseases are closely related to the patient's emotional state. Numerous scientific studies show that most patients suffering from gastroesophageal reflux also suffer from anxiety or depression. It is therefore recommended to consider these factors in the choice of treatment plan. The psychological treatment plan consists of cognitive-behavioral therapy, which is extremely effective in managing anxiety.

12.6 Conclusions

In conclusion, the management of patients with esophageal diseases requires a multidisciplinary approach involving the collaboration of a doctor, a surgeon, a physiotherapist, a nutritionist, and a psychotherapist, to successfully improve the patient's quality of life, especially in the long term.

References

1. De Troyer A, Sampson M, Sigrist S, Macklem PT. The diaphragm: two muscles. Science. 1981;213(4504):237–8.
2. Mittal RK. The crural diaphragm, an external lower esophageal sphincter: a definitive study. Gastroenterology. 1993;105:1565–7.
3. Kahrilas PJ, Mittal RK, Bor S, et al. Chicago Classification update (v4.0): technical review of high-resolution manometry metrics for EGJ barrier function. Neurogastroenterol Motil. 2021;33(10):e14113.
4. Zdrhova L, Bitnar P, Balihar K, et al. Breathing exercise in gastroesophageal reflux disease: a systematic review. Dysphagia. 2023;38(2):609–21.
5. Siboni S, Bonavina L, Rogers BD, et al. Effect of increased intra-abdominal pressure on the esophagogastric junction: a systematic review. J Clin Gastroenterol. 2022;56(10):821–30.
6. Trabucco I. Stop al reflusso con il metodo Trabucco. Independently published; 2018.

Open Access This chapter is licensed under the terms of the Creative Commons Attribution-NonCommercial 4.0 International License (http://creativecommons.org/licenses/by-nc/4.0/), which permits any noncommercial use, sharing, adaptation, distribution and reproduction in any medium or format, as long as you give appropriate credit to the original author(s) and the source, provide a link to the Creative Commons license and indicate if changes were made.

The images or other third party material in this chapter are included in the chapter's Creative Commons license, unless indicated otherwise in a credit line to the material. If material is not included in the chapter's Creative Commons license and your intended use is not permitted by statutory regulation or exceeds the permitted use, you will need to obtain permission directly from the copyright holder.

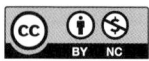

Surgical Antireflux Procedures

13

Vincenzo Landolfi and Salvatore Tolone

13.1 Introduction

Gastroesophageal reflux disease (GERD) is a prevalent health condition. As of 2020, the global prevalence of GERD was recorded at 13.98% [1]. When symptoms and/or complications of GERD are present, the mainstay treatment is represented by the administration of proton-pump inhibitors (PPIs) with or without the addition of prokinetics, antacids, or newly developed potassium-competitive acid blockers (PCABs) or topical mucosal defensive agents. On the other hand, GERD can also be treated using antireflux surgery (ARS), which may be indicated in the presence of "proven" GERD and usually when the patient is considered truly refractory to medical therapy [2]. However, ARS may also be indicated when a patient with "proven" GERD is not willing to continue life-long therapy. The term "proven GERD" refers to a clinical condition in which the presence of pathological reflux is objectively demonstrated (e.g., mucosal damage observed through endoscopic examination and/or abnormal acid exposure in the esophagus during pH monitoring). Furthermore, the Lyon Consensus 2.0 introduced the new relevant concept of "actionable GERD" [3]. This means that in the presence of troublesome proven GERD, therapeutic options including surgery should be initiated. According to the 2021 guidelines from the American College of Gastroenterology (ACG) [4], an 8-week, once-daily empirical PPI therapy is recommended for patients with typical GERD symptoms who do not exhibit alarming signs such as weight loss or gastrointestinal bleeding. However, nearly 40% of patients on PPI therapy continue to

V. Landolfi
UOC General Surgery, AORN San Giuseppe Moscati, Avellino, Italy
e-mail: vincenzo.landolfi@aornmoscati.it

S. Tolone (✉)
UOC General, Mininvasive, Oncological and Bariatric Surgery,
University of Campania "Luigi Vanvitelli", Naples, Italy
e-mail: salvatore.tolone@unicampania.it

© The Author(s) 2026
V. Landolfi, S. Tolone (eds.), *Functional Diseases of the Esophagus*, Updates in Surgery, https://doi.org/10.1007/978-3-031-90570-4_13

experience symptoms like heartburn and regurgitation [5]. Refractory GERD is generally defined by persistent heartburn or regurgitation even after 8 to 12 weeks of double-dose PPI therapy. Observational studies have linked long-term PPI use to various adverse effects, including dementia, osteoporosis, pneumonia, and *Clostridium difficile* infection. ARS has shown comparable or even greater effectiveness to medications, including PPIs, as shown by a meta-analysis of randomized controlled trials (RCTs) [6]. Consequently, the ACG guidelines recommend ARS as a long-term treatment for individuals with severe reflux esophagitis (Los Angeles grade C or D), large hiatal hernias, or ongoing troublesome GERD symptoms that are confirmed through objective testing.

GERD is frequently linked to hiatal hernia, a condition in which the esophagogastric junction (EGJ) and a portion of the stomach herniate through the esophageal hiatus. In these cases, the lower esophageal sphincter (LES) is displaced upward, disturbing the balance between the intrinsic LES pressure and the external compression exerted by the diaphragmatic crura, and thus reducing LES pressure. Current guidelines advocate for the surgical repair of symptomatic hiatal hernias, a process that usually includes primary crural closure, with or without reinforcement with a mesh, and ARS [7].

Moreover, the 2021 guidelines from the Society of American Gastrointestinal and Endoscopic Surgeons indicate that ARS might be more effective than medical management for patients with chronic or treatment-resistant GERD. This recommendation is supported by evidence of four favorable outcomes: a reduction in the time the pH remains below 4, a decreased dependency on PPIs after the procedure, improvements in short-term quality of life, and more effective long-term symptom control. Although potential adverse effects such as short-term complications, gas, bloating, and occasional treatment failures may occur, these risks are generally considered minor when weighed against the benefits.

13.2 Mechanisms of Efficacy of Antireflux Surgery

ARS started more than half a century ago, when Nissen wrapped the gastric fundus to protect an esophagogastric anastomosis after a cardia resection for cancer and subsequently noted the absence of pathological reflux exposure in the patient. The Nissen fundoplication was subsequently perfected and used with optimal results. Then Mario Rossetti described his variant of total fundoplication (Nissen-Rossetti fundoplication, Fig. 13.1), whereas Toupet (Fig. 13.2) and Dor described their technique of partial posterior and partial anterior fundoplication, respectively. Finally, DeMeester and Donahue described their concept of a "floppy Nissen" fundoplication.

All these techniques have in common the same principle: to create a new mechanical barrier by wrapping the fundus around the EGJ. However, it is fundamental to keep in mind that ARS is not only "fashioning a wrap", but it is an anatomical restoration of the EGJ. In fact, all ARS procedures need careful preparation of the diaphragmatic pillars, a long mediastinal esophageal preparation to obtain an

Fig. 13.1 Laparoscopic Nissen-Rossetti fundoplication. (Courtesy of Prof S. Tolone)

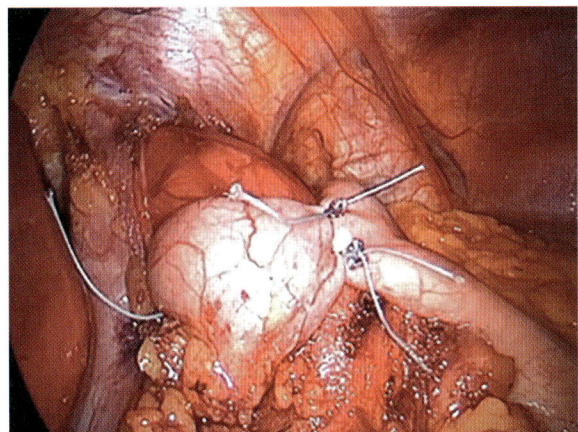

Fig. 13.2 Laparoscopic Toupet fundoplication. (Courtesy of Prof S. Tolone)

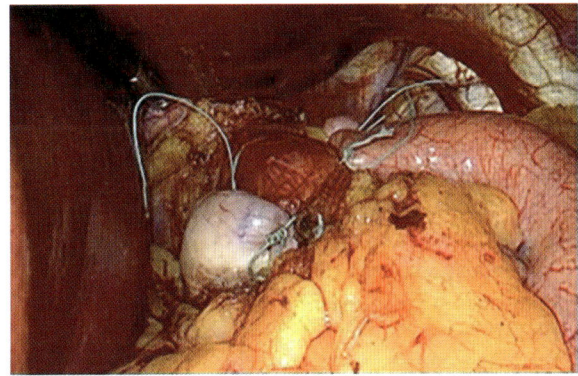

adequate intrabdominal segment (without traction, or floppy), preservation of the anterior and posterior vagal nerves, and adequate closure of the hiatal defect (with or without meshes). Finally, the fundoplication should be fashioned exactly around the EGJ, because a wrap that is too proximal can expose the distal esophageal mucosa to reflux, and one that is too distal can similarly expose to reflux and can also increase postoperative dysphagia. Achieving all these key aspects during ARS ensures that the EGJ pressure is increased and transient lower esophageal sphincter relaxations are reduced (because of the wrap and the crural functions), and the hiatal hernia is resolved. Thus, this mechanical barrier has been proved effective in controlling all kinds of reflux (acid, weakly acid and weakly alkaline), as well as relieving all the symptoms directly related to the reflux and stopping the damaging action of the gastric contents on the esophageal mucosa [8].

Given these features, ARS has been shown to result in a drastic relief of symptoms and complications in individuals diagnosed with "proven" GERD who respond poorly to PPIs, as demonstrated by a recent RCT by Spechler et al. [9]. The procedure notably decreases both the duration of acid exposure in the esophagus and the number of reflux events, leading to complete or partial symptom remission within 3 months after surgery. On the other hand, when GERD is not demonstrated, as in patients with functional esophageal disorders or in those considered to have reflux hypersensitivity, the use of ARS is debated because, although it has shown positive effects in symptom reduction, the supporting evidence remains limited [10], and individuals who do not respond well to PPI treatment may also achieve less-than-optimal symptom relief following ARS [11]. For example, Wilkerson et al. [12] observed considerable symptom improvement after surgery in both PPI responders and non-responders, although the responders experienced slightly better outcomes (94% vs. 87%; p = 0.08). Similarly, another prospective study demonstrated that while the anatomical outcomes after ARS were similar for both groups, symptom remission was significantly higher among responders (heartburn: 93% vs. 73%, p = 0.01; regurgitation: 96% vs. 84%, p = 0.04; atypical symptoms, such as asthma, chest pain, or cough: 96.6% vs. 83.9%, p = 0.002) [11]. These differences could be attributed to the presence of undiagnosed functional esophageal disorders in some patients, highlighting the need to distinguish these conditions from GERD using diagnostic tools such as endoscopy, esophageal pH monitoring, assessment of acid exposure time, and calculation of the DeMeester score.

ARS is a valuable treatment option for managing refractory GERD, offering promising results and cost-effectiveness. However, meticulous patient selection is essential, particularly because ARS tends to be less effective in PPI non-responders, is irreversible, and carries the risk of postoperative complications. Spechler et al.'s landmark study demonstrated that, when GERD is accurately diagnosed using upper endoscopy, high-resolution manometry, and pH-monitoring or pH-impedance monitoring, ARS is markedly superior to PPI therapy in patients with refractory GERD [9].

Historically, the guidelines have supported ARS as an alternative for patients who require continuous PPI therapy, especially those with abnormal esophageal acid exposure as evidenced by 24-hour monitoring studies. This recommendation applies to both erosive reflux disease and non-erosive reflux disease, provided that esophageal motility disorders have been ruled out by manometry. More recent research indicates that ARS might also be advantageous for patients with reflux hypersensitivity—defined by a high symptom index (>50%) or a symptom-associated probability exceeding 95%—which reflects a strong correlation between symptoms and reflux events, even in the absence of a formal GERD diagnosis [8].

Meta-analyses of RCTs comparing ARS with PPI therapy in confirmed GERD patients generally indicate that ARS provides equal or superior symptom management, although the incidence of posttreatment complications is similar or, in some instances, slightly higher with surgery. For example, Tristão et al. found that fundoplication resulted in a significantly greater remission of heartburn (risk difference [RD]: −0.19, p = 0.0003) while achieving comparable outcomes for the remission of regurgitation (RD: −0.07, p = 0.18), abnormal esophageal acid exposure (pH <4) (mean difference [MD]: −2.40, p = 0.64), and the frequency of dysphagia and other complications when compared to PPI treatment [6]. Similarly, research by Garg et al. demonstrated that both short- and long-term postoperative heartburn and other reflux symptoms were less common among ARS patients than those on PPIs, and that ARS patients enjoyed improved health-related quality of life scores (short-term standardized mean difference [SMD] 0.14, 95% CI −0.02 to 0.03). However, this benefit was counterbalanced by a higher occurrence of short-term dysphagia (RR 3.58, 95% CI 1.91 to 6.71) and serious adverse events (RR 1.46, 95% CI 1.01 to 2.11) following surgery [13].

Limited studies suggest that patients with reflux hypersensitivity or other functional esophageal disorders, may also benefit from ARS. For example, one RCT reported that 1 year after ARS, 71% of patients with reflux hypersensitivity experienced symptom improvement, compared to 62% of patients with standard GERD and only 12% in the placebo group [14].

13.3 Which Kind of Fundoplication Should Be Chosen?

Nissen fundoplication is the most widely performed procedure in ARS, although partial fundoplication (Dor and Toupet) methods are also used to lessen the risk of postoperative dysphagia, bloating, and other complications.

Meta-analyses of RCTs comparing Nissen and Dor fundoplication reveal that the Nissen procedure is associated with a higher incidence of postoperative dysphagia (RR 0.56, $p = 0.002$), flatulence (RR 0.57, $p = 0.02$), inability to belch (RR 0.63, $p = 0.05$), and gas bloating (RR 0.59, $p < 0.001$) than the Dor approach. However, there were no significant differences between the two procedures regarding postoperative heartburn (RR 1.39, $p = 0.58$) or the continued use of PPIs. Additionally, measures such as postoperative DeMeester scores (weighted mean difference [WMD] 0.85, $p = 0.06$), LES pressure (SMD $−0.74$ mmHg, $p = 0.23$), and reoperation rates (RR 1.50, $p = 0.24$) were similar between the groups [15].

Similarly, comparisons between Nissen and Toupet fundoplication indicate that patients undergoing the Nissen procedure may experience higher rates of postoperative dysphagia (RR 2.61, $p < 0.01$) and gas-related symptoms (RR 1.31, $p = 0.02$), including difficulties with belching, gas bloating, and flatulence. Although patient satisfaction (RR 1.05, $p = 0.22$) and reoperation rates (4.74% vs. 6.54%, $p = 0.77$) were comparable, the Nissen technique resulted in higher postoperative LES pressure (SMD 0.66, $p < 0.05$) and a lower, though not statistically significant, postoperative DeMeester score (SMD $−0.72$, $p = 0.06$) relative to Toupet fundoplication [16]. However, more recent studies showed no systematic discrepancy between the Nissen and Toupet fundoplication for intraoperative complications (Nissen 2.10% vs. Toupet 1.48%), general complications (2.27% vs. 2.88%), postoperative complications (1.44% vs. 1.18%), complication-related reoperation (1.00% vs. 0.91%), recurrence at 1-year follow-up (6.55% vs. 5.33%), pain on exertion at 1-year follow-up (12.49% vs. 9.52%), pain at rest at 1-year follow-up (10.44 vs. 9.52%) and pain requiring treatment at 1-year follow-up (9.61% vs. 8.17%). Also the postoperative dysphagia rate was 5.34% after Nissen and 4.64% after Toupet, with no significant difference [17].

In summary, while Nissen fundoplication may provide superior control of reflux symptoms, it is also associated with a higher risk of postoperative issues such as dysphagia and gas bloating. Recent guidelines suggest that the choice of surgical approach should be tailored to the patient's priorities –whether they favor maximal symptom relief or wish to minimize potential postoperative side effects like dysphagia. However, we would highlight that it is fundamental for a surgeon dedicated to ARS to be confident with all kinds of fundoplication, in order to offer the best option for the single patient.

13.4 Laparoscopic or Robot-Assisted ARS?

With the advent of robotic surgery, many authors claimed that robotic antireflux surgery (RARS) can present better outcomes, fewer complications and shorter hospital stays, paying the price for a more expensive technology and a longer operative time. According to a recent systematic review and meta-analysis, the results of laparoscopic ARS vs. RARS showed no statistically significant difference in operative time, intraoperative complications, length of stay, readmission rates, overall complications, and mortality. However, laparoscopic ARS was associated with lower costs compared to RARS [18]. These results seem to be intuitive, because the cost of a new technology is always more expensive at the start, with an obvious decrease in time, as the history of laparoscopy has just taught us. The key issue is to continue providing a standardized ARS with its principles, whether via laparoscopy or robot-assisted laparoscopy.

13.5 New Technologies

The history of ARS is constellated with many attempts to use alternative devices to fundoplication, such as the old Angelchik prosthesis, implantable agents, electrical pacemakers and endoscopic techniques. However, only magnetic sphincter augmentation by means of a ring device constituted by several magnetic beads (LINX™, J&J) is currently used in clinical practice. Current indications are the same as for ARS, with the only limitation of placing the device in patients with a still adequate esophageal motility (mean distal esophageal amplitude >30 mmHg). The ring diameter is chosen intraoperatively, with a dedicated calibrating device; the magnetic sphincter is placed around the LES passing between the posterior vagus and the esophageal wall. Its unique feature is that it expands by separating the beads when a pressure greater than 30 mmHg is applied. Thus, food is allowed to pass reducing the probability of postoperative dysphagia, gas-bloat syndrome and inability to belch and vomiting, but effectively controlling the reflux that is known to occur through a low pressure system. Outcome data after at least 5 years of follow-up showed optimal reflux control, low PPI resumption rate and a 4% rate of device removal [19, 20].

13.6 Conclusion

ARS is an effective and safe treatment for GERD. The most important requisite is to provide objective evidence of GERD and to accurately select the patient using objective testing. Each type of fundoplication has its place in the surgical management of GERD, offering unique benefits based on patient-specific factors such as esophageal motility, symptom severity, and anatomical considerations. The choice of procedure should be guided by a thorough preoperative evaluation to optimize patient outcomes, with careful consideration given to long-term outcomes and potential complications. As laparoscopic fundoplication techniques evolve, the trend toward patient-specific approaches and minimally invasive technology is anticipated to further refine the effectiveness and durability of surgical interventions for GERD.

References

1. Nirwan JS, Hasan SS, Babar ZU, et al. Global prevalence and risk factors of gastro-oesophageal reflux disease (GORD): systematic review with meta-analysis. Sci Rep. 2020;10:5814.
2. Gensthaler L, Schoppmann SF. New developments in anti-reflux surgery: where are we now? Visc Med. 2024;40(5):250–5.
3. Gyawali CP, Yadlapati R, Fass R, et al. Updates to the modern diagnosis of GERD: Lyon consensus 2.0. Gut. 2024;73(2):361–71.
4. Katz PO, Dunbar KB, Schnoll-Sussman FH, et al. ACG clinical guideline for the diagnosis and management of gastroesophageal reflux disease. Am J Gastroenterol. 2022;117:27–56.
5. El-Serag H, Becher A, Jones R. Systematic review: persistent reflux symptoms on proton pump inhibitor therapy in primary care and community studies. Aliment Pharmacol Ther. 2010;32:720–37.
6. Tristão LS, Tustumi F, Tavares G, Bernardo WM. Fundoplication versus oral proton pump inhibitors for gastroesophageal reflux disease: a systematic review and meta-analysis of randomized clinical trials. Esophagus. 2021;18:173–80.
7. Pauwels A, Boecxstaens V, Andrews CN, et al. How to select patients for antireflux surgery? The ICARUS guidelines (international consensus regarding preoperative examinations and clinical characteristics assessment to select adult patients for antireflux surgery). Gut. 2019;68:1928–41.
8. del Genio G, Tolone S, del Genio F, et al. Prospective assessment of patient selection for antireflux surgery by combined multichannel intraluminal impedance pH monitoring. J Gastrointest Surg. 2008;12(9):1491–6.
9. Spechler SJ, Hunter JG, Jones KM, et al. Randomized trial of medical versus surgical treatment for refractory heartburn. N Engl J Med. 2019;381:1513–23.
10. Lee I, Park S. Diagnosis and treatment of reflux hypersensitivity with gastroesophageal reflux symptoms from a surgical perspective. Foregut Surg. 2022;2:8–16.
11. Morgenthal CB, Lin E, Shane MD, et al. Who will fail laparoscopic Nissen fundoplication? Preoperative prediction of long-term outcomes. Surg Endosc. 2007;21:1978–84.
12. Wilkerson PM, Stratford J, Jones L, et al. A poor response to proton pump inhibition is not a contraindication for laparoscopic antireflux surgery for gastro esophageal reflux disease. Surg Endosc. 2005;19:1272–7.
13. Garg SK, Gurusamy KS. Laparoscopic fundoplication surgery versus medical management for gastro-oesophageal reflux disease (GORD) in adults. Cochrane Database Syst Rev. 2015;2015:CD003243.

14. Mainie I, Tutuian R, Agrawal A, et al. Combined multichannel intraluminal impedance-pH monitoring to select patients with persistent gastro-oesophageal reflux for laparoscopic Nissen fundoplication. Br J Surg. 2006;93:1483–7.
15. Raue W, Ordemann J, Jacobi CA, et al. Nissen versus dor fundoplication for treatment of gastroesophageal reflux disease: a blinded randomized clinical trial. Dig Surg. 2011;28(1):80–6.
16. Tian ZC, Wang B, Shan CX, et al. A meta-analysis of randomized controlled trials to compare long-term outcomes of Nissen and Toupet fundoplication for gastroesophageal reflux disease. PLoS One. 2015;10(6):e0127627.
17. Köckerling F, Jacob D, Adolf D, et al. Laparoscopic total (Nissen) versus posterior (Toupet) fundoplication for gastroesophageal reflux disease: a propensity score-matched comparison of the perioperative and 1-year follow-up outcome. Hernia. 2024;28(5):1629–39.
18. Gonçalves-Costa D, Barbosa JP, Quesado R, et al. Robotic surgery versus laparoscopic surgery for anti-reflux and hiatal hernia surgery: a short-term outcomes and cost systematic literature review and meta-analysis. Langenbeck's Arch Surg. 2024;409(1):175.
19. Fadel MG, Tarazi M, Dave M, et al. Magnetic sphincter augmentation in the management of gastro-esophageal reflux disease: a systematic review and meta-analysis. Int J Surg. 2024;110(10):6355–66.
20. Bonavina L, Horbach T, Schoppmann SF, DeMarchi J. Three-year clinical experience with magnetic sphincter augmentation and laparoscopic fundoplication. Surg Endosc. 2021;35(7):3449–58.

Open Access This chapter is licensed under the terms of the Creative Commons Attribution-NonCommercial 4.0 International License (http://creativecommons.org/licenses/by-nc/4.0/), which permits any noncommercial use, sharing, adaptation, distribution and reproduction in any medium or format, as long as you give appropriate credit to the original author(s) and the source, provide a link to the Creative Commons license and indicate if changes were made.

The images or other third party material in this chapter are included in the chapter's Creative Commons license, unless indicated otherwise in a credit line to the material. If material is not included in the chapter's Creative Commons license and your intended use is not permitted by statutory regulation or exceeds the permitted use, you will need to obtain permission directly from the copyright holder.

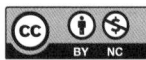

Endoscopic Treatment of Gastroesophageal Reflux Disease

Guido Costamagna and Cristina Ciuffini

14.1 Introduction

Gastroesophageal reflux disease (GERD) is one of the most common chronic conditions affecting the upper digestive system [1]. GERD occurs when the backward flow of stomach contents into the esophagus causes symptoms and/or mucosal injuries [2]. The primary pathophysiological mechanisms of GERD are lower esophageal sphincter (LES) dysfunction and impaired esophageal motility that are responsible for the upflow and persistence of gastric contents in the esophagus, respectively [2]. Typical symptoms include heartburn and regurgitation, but GERD can also present through atypical or extra-esophageal symptoms such as laryngitis, asthma and cough [2]. The presence of symptoms without mucosal damage is defined as "non-erosive reflux disease" (NERD) [2]. Conversely, patients with evidence of esophageal mucosal breaks at endoscopy are diagnosed with erosive esophagitis and have an increased risk of developing complications like esophageal ulcers and strictures, Barrett's esophagus, and esophageal adenocarcinoma [2]. Traditional treatments include lifestyle modifications, pharmacologic therapy, and surgical interventions [3]. Proton-pump inhibitors (PPIs) are the most commonly used medication and have proven to be effective in providing symptom relief and promoting mucosal healing [3]. However, many patients experience a symptomatic relapse and the recurrence of erosive esophagitis upon discontinuation of therapy [3]. On the other hand, long-term PPI therapy has raised growing concern about the side effects, especially the increased risk of infections and malabsorption [4]. Additionally, some patients exhibit PPI-refractory GERD, which is defined as the persistence of typical symptoms after 8 weeks of double-dose PPI therapy [3]. Surgical intervention is a valid option for PPI-refractory or PPI-dependent patients

G. Costamagna (✉) · C. Ciuffini
Centre of Excellence for Gastrointestinal and Endocrine-Metabolic Diseases,
Digestive Endoscopy Unit, Ospedale Isola Tiberina – Gemelli Isola, Rome, Italy
e-mail: guido.costamagna@fbf-isola.it; cristina.ciuffini.fw@fbf-isola.it

[3]. Nevertheless, antireflux surgery, primarily fundoplication, carries a risk of acute complications [5]. Since the early 2000s, the development of endoscopic treatments offers minimally invasive alternatives with promising efficacy and safety profiles for patients with GERD who are refractory to medical therapy, those who are not candidates for surgery, or those preferring a less invasive approach [6]. General contraindications to endoscopic therapy for GERD include the presence of a hiatal hernia larger than 2 cm, severe erosive esophagitis, esophageal strictures, and Barrett's esophagus [6]. This chapter will discuss the main endoscopic techniques, their mechanisms of action, and their clinical outcomes.

14.2 Types of Endoscopic Treatments

Injection of bulking agents. Early efforts in endoscopic treatment of GERD involved injecting bulking agents at the esophagogastric junction (EGJ) to improve its antireflux barrier function [7, 8]. Despite early promise, these products have been withdrawn or sidelined, and none are currently approved for clinical practice. Enteryx is a biocompatible non-resorbable copolymer that is injected in the muscle layer where it solidifies into a spongy mass [7]. An international multicenter prospective trial demonstrated that PPI cessation persisted in 67% of patients after 24 months of Enteryx implantation [9]. Despite this, Enteryx was withdrawn from the market in 2005 due to safety concerns after reports of mediastinal complications [7, 9, 10]. A similar fate befell the Gatekeeper reflux repair system, consisting of expandable hydrogel prostheses implanted into the submucosa of the LES area, that was able to significantly improve GERD health-related quality of life (GERD-HRQL) and normalize esophageal pH [8]. However, the Gatekeeper reflux repair system is no longer marketed due to the lack of long-term results. Later on, other bulking agents, such as Durasphere and Plexiglas, showed initial success in small studies but were not pursued in further trials [11, 12].

Radiofrequency energy treatment (STRETTA® procedure). The STRETTA® procedure was first approved by the FDA for the treatment of GERD in 2000 and is the endoscopic technique with the most extensive clinical experience to date [13, 14]. It involves the delivery of low-power radiofrequency energy using four needle electrodes that extend from a balloon catheter into the muscle layer at different levels across the LES and the gastric cardia [15]. Although the exact mechanism of action remains unclear, it is hypothesized that radiofrequency stimulation thickens the LES wall through fibrosis and muscle hypertrophy [16, 17]. A 2017 meta-analysis of the STRETTA® procedure demonstrated significant improvements in HRQL scores and a marked decrease in heartburn symptoms [14]. Of all patients, 51% discontinued PPIs, while 36% exhibited significant healing of erosive esophagitis at follow-up endoscopy [14]. The safety profile of the procedure was excellent, with an adverse event rate of less than 1% [14]. Erosion and mucosal lacerations were the most common complication [14]. Several longer-term follow-up studies have shown that the STRETTA® procedure yields sustained improvements in heartburn scores, patient satisfaction, and reduced PPI use, with positive outcomes reported up to 4, 8, and even 10 years after the procedure [18–20].

Transoral incisionless fundoplication. Transoral incisionless fundoplication (TIF) using the EsophyX™, approved by the FDA in 2007, allows the gastric fundus to be wrapped around the lower esophagus without the need for external incisions [6]. The procedure involves two endoscopists: one handles the gastroscope, which is positioned retroflexed to view the cardia, while the other operates the EsophyX™ device, which is loaded onto a gastroscope and introduced transorally under direct vision [6]. A helical retractor is inserted into the EGJ tissue with a corkscrew-like motion to pull the tissue down and create a fold that is secured in place with two small fasteners [6]. The process is repeated around the EGJ until a valve 2 to 4 cm in length and 270 to 300 degrees in circumference is achieved [6] (Fig. 14.1). The flap valve's luminal diameter is controlled by the device, preventing over-tightening and allowing intragastric air to vent [21]. This minimizes the onset of dysphagia and gas-related symptoms, common sequelae of conventional antireflux surgery [21]. TIF is the most extensively researched plication device for GERD, supported by several well-conducted meta-analyses demonstrating its effectiveness. Overall, TIF proved to be able to improve HRQL and typical symptoms as well as atypical ones with discontinuation of PPI in almost 90% of patients [22–24]. These results are durable, with over 90% of patients having reduced their PPI use by more than 50% in a 10-year follow-up study [25]. The procedure also showed a good safety profile with a 1–2% rate of adverse events [22, 24].

Another system developed to create a partial endoscopic fundoplication is the Medigus Ultrasonic Surgical Endostapler (MUSE™) that was cleared by FDA in

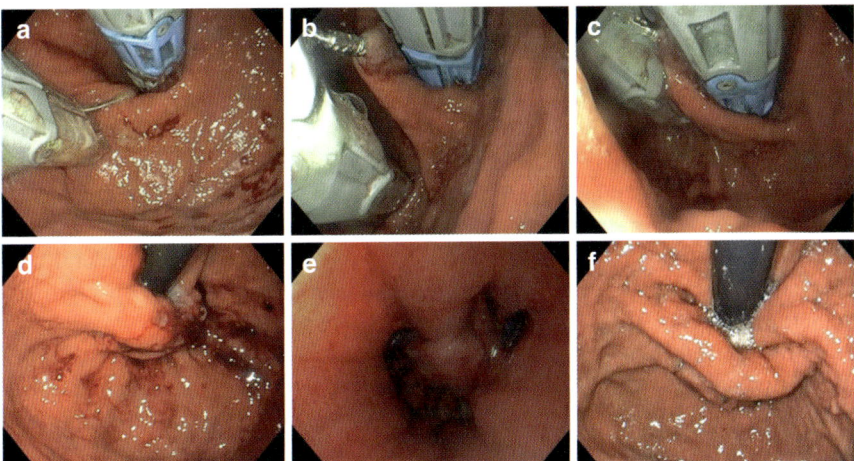

Fig. 14.1 Transoral incisionless fundoplication (TIF) with EsophyX™. (**a**) A helical retractor is inserted into the EGJ tissue with a corkscrew-like motion. (**b**) The tissue is pulled down between the arms of the device. (**c**) The fold is secured in place with fasteners. (**d**) Appearance of the cardia in retroflexed position at the end of the procedure. (**e**) Appearance of the cardia in anterovision at the end of the procedure. (**f**) Appearance of the cardia in retrovision at the 6-month follow-up

2015 [6]. The endostapler, which resembles an endoscope, is introduced into the stomach through an overtube [6]. The endoscope tip is then retroflexed and maneuvered to align the anvil with the rigid section of the endoscope shaft, which contains the staple cartridge [6]. This positioning, approximately 3 cm proximal to the EGJ, allows the tissue of the fundus to be clamped against the distal esophagus where it is secured by firing staples [6]. An ultrasound device is located at the tip of the endostapler [6]. It uses an ultrasonic range finder to measure the tissue gap and alignment between the staple cartridge and the anvil, displaying this information on a video monitor [6]. The MUSE™ device is rotated, and the procedure is repeated to achieve a 180-degree anterior fundoplication [6]. In a multicentre, prospective trial 83.8% of patients remained off daily PPI at 6 months after procedure, with 69.4% still off at 4 years [26]. Additionally, GERD-HRQL showed a significant increase from baseline to both 6 months and 4 years after the procedure [26]. Initially, safety concerns emerged following serious adverse events including severe upper GI bleeding and esophageal leakage [27, 28]. However, after the introduction of protocol measures such as antiemetic prophylaxis and postoperative X-rays, no further severe adverse events were reported [26]. Unfortunately, the MUSE™ system is not being merchandized at the moment following company-specific issues.

Endoscopic full-thickness plication. The NDO full-thickness plicator was developed in the early 2000s to create full-thickness plications at the EGJ [29]. In this procedure, the endoscope/plicator assembly is introduced in the stomach and placed in retroflex position [30]. A helical tissue retractor is inserted deep into the gastric wall, within 1 cm below the EGJ [30]. The gastric wall is then drawn between the arms of the plicator, which are subsequently closed to deploy a suture, securing the full-thickness plication [30]. The NDO plicator procedure proved to be safe and effective in reducing GERD symptoms and the need for medication, with its effects demonstrating long-term durability for up to 5 years [31]. However, it was withdrawn from the market in 2008 due to the company's financial difficulties [29]. Subsequently, an improved and redesigned version of the plicator, the GERDx™, was introduced. In a 2018 study by Weitzendorfer et al., endoscopic full-thickness plication with the GERDx™ device effectively reduced esophageal acid exposure and medication use, relieved reflux-related symptoms, and improved patients' HRQL [32]. However, four serious adverse events were reported, including a EGJ hematoma, pneumonia, a Mallory-Weiss lesion, and severe post-procedural pain requiring surgical removal of a suture that had passed through the diaphragm and the left hepatic lobe [32]. These complications were ascribed to temporary changes in the material and length of the sutures, and no adverse events were observed when the original sutures were used [32, 33]. In a subsequent randomized, sham-controlled study involving PPI-dependent patients, endoscopic full-thickness plication with the GERDx™ device proved to be both safe and effective, showing a gradual improvement in typical symptoms and GERD-HRQL scores at 3, 6, and 12 months [34]. After 12 months, 62.8% of patients in the GERDx™ group were off PPIs, with no major adverse events reported [34].

Antireflux mucosectomy and mucosal ablation. Antireflux mucosectomy (ARMS), first described by Inoue et al. in 2014, involves a hemicircumferential endoscopic mucosal resection of the gastric cardia [35]. The concept of ARMS arose from the observation that patients who underwent circumferential mucosal resection for Barrett's esophagus with high-grade dysplasia showed an improvement in GERD symptoms [35]. It was hypothesized that scar formation after the mucosal defect healed would cause a narrowing of the cardia [35]. A 2022 meta-analysis of 10 studies involving 307 patients showed that ARMS significantly improved GERD-HRQL scores and resulted in a 65.3% rate of discontinuation and a 21.5% reduction in PPI use [36]. However, the procedure was associated with a 17.2% adverse event rate, with dysphagia from esophageal stricture being the most common complication [36]. In 2020, Inoue et al. introduced a newer technique called antireflux mucosal ablation (ARMA), which offers the advantage of being repeatable regardless of the presence of fibrosis [37]. The procedure involves ablating the mucosa around the cardia using an endoscopic knife connected to an electrocautery generator set to coagulation mode, or, more recently, an argon plasma coagulation probe [37, 38]). The ablation is performed with the endoscope in a retroflexed position on the gastric side, while preserving two contralateral mucosal areas to prevent stenosis [37, 38]. In a 2024 bi-center study involving 68 patients, ARMA demonstrated to be a straightforward, safe, and effective procedure able to improve GERD-HRQL and reduce esophageal acid exposure and erosive esophagitis [38]). The most frequently reported adverse events were dysphagia requiring endoscopic balloon dilation in 13.2% of cases, and mild to moderate delayed bleeding in 8.8% of cases [38].

14.3 Conclusion

Endoscopic techniques have emerged as a promising and innovative approach for the treatment of selected patients with GERD, demonstrating both efficacy and safety. However, these procedures are highly specialized and require significant technical expertise to perform correctly. Consequently, at this time, they should be reserved for application in specialized tertiary care centers. Further research and continued refinement of the devices will be pivotal to expand their availability and accessibility, potentially offering new therapeutic options for a broader patient population in the future.

References

1. Li N, Yang WL, Cai MH, et al. Burden of gastroesophageal reflux disease in 204 countries and territories, 1990–2019: a systematic analysis for the global burden of disease study 2019. BMC Public Health. 2023;23(1):582.
2. Moayyedi P, Talley NJ. Gastro-oesophageal reflux disease. Lancet. 2006;367(9528):2086–100.
3. Katz PO, Dunbar KB, Schnoll-Sussman FH, et al. ACG clinical guideline for the diagnosis and management of gastroesophageal reflux disease. Am J Gastroenterol. 2022;117(1):27–56.
4. Haastrup PF, Thompson W, Søndergaard J, Jarbøl DE. Side effects of long-term proton pump inhibitor use: a review. Basic Clin Pharma Tox. 2018;123(2):114–21.

5. Maret-Ouda J, Wahlin K, El-Serag HB, Lagergren J. Association between laparoscopic antireflux surgery and recurrence of gastroesophageal reflux. JAMA. 2017;318(10):939–46.
6. Technology Committee ASGE, Thosani N, Goodman A, et al. Endoscopic anti-reflux devices (with videos). Gastrointest Endosc. 2017 Dec;86(6):931–48.
7. Devière J, Costamagna G, Neuhaus H, et al. Nonresorbable copolymer implantation for gastroesophageal reflux disease: a randomized sham-controlled multicenter trial. Gastroenterology. 2005;128(3):532–40.
8. Fockens P, Bruno MJ, Gabbrielli A, et al. Endoscopic augmentation of the lower esophageal sphincter for the treatment of gastroesophageal reflux disease: multicenter study of the gatekeeper reflux repair system. Endoscopy. 2004;36(8):682–9.
9. Cohen LB, Johnson DA, Ganz RA, et al. Enteryx implantation for GERD: expanded multicenter trial results and interim postapproval follow-up to 24 months. Gastrointest Endosc. 2005;61(6):650–8.
10. Wong RF, Davis TV, Peterson KA. Complications involving the mediastinum after injection of Enteryx for GERD. Gastrointest Endosc. 2005;61(6):753–6.
11. Ganz RA, Fallon E, Wittchow T, Klein D. A new injectable agent for the treatment of GERD: results of the Durasphere pilot trial. Gastrointest Endosc. 2009;69(2):318–23.
12. Feretis C, Benakis P, Dimopoulos C, et al. Endoscopic implantation of Plexiglas (PMMA) microspheres for the treatment of GERD. Gastrointest Endosc. 2001;53(4):423–6.
13. Guidelines Committee SAGES, Auyang ED, Carter P, et al. SAGES clinical spotlight review: endoluminal treatments for gastroesophageal reflux disease (GERD). Surg Endosc. 2013;27(8):2658–72.
14. Fass R, Cahn F, Scotti DJ, Gregory DA. Systematic review and meta-analysis of controlled and prospective cohort efficacy studies of endoscopic radiofrequency for treatment of gastroesophageal reflux disease. Surg Endosc. 2017;31(12):4865–82.
15. Triadafilopoulos G, DiBaise JK, Nostrant TT, et al. Radiofrequency energy delivery to the gastroesophageal junction for the treatment of GERD. Gastrointest Endosc. 2001;53(4):407–15.
16. Kim MS, Holloway RH, Dent J, Utley DS. Radiofrequency energy delivery to the gastric cardia inhibits triggering of transient lower esophageal sphincter relaxation and gastroesophageal reflux in dogs. Gastrointest Endosc. 2003;57(1):17–22.
17. Tam WCE. Delivery of radiofrequency energy to the lower oesophageal sphincter and gastric cardia inhibits transient lower oesophageal sphincter relaxations and gastro-oesophageal reflux in patients with reflux disease. Gut. 2003;52(4):479–85.
18. Reymunde A, Santiago N. Long-term results of radiofrequency energy delivery for the treatment of GERD: sustained improvements in symptoms, quality of life, and drug use at 4-year follow-up. Gastrointest Endosc. 2007;65(3):361–6.
19. Dughera L, Rotondano G, De Cento M, et al. Durability of Stretta radiofrequency treatment for GERD: results of an 8-year follow-up. Gastroenterol Res Pract. 2014;2014:531907.
20. Noar M, Squires P, Noar E, Lee M. Long-term maintenance effect of radiofrequency energy delivery for refractory GERD: a decade later. Surg Endosc. 2014;28(8):2323–33.
21. Rinsma NF, Smeets FG, Bruls DW, et al. Effect of transoral incisionless fundoplication on reflux mechanisms. Surg Endosc. 2014;28(3):941–9.
22. McCarty T, Itidiare M, Njei B, Rustagi T. Efficacy of transoral incisionless fundoplication for refractory gastroesophageal reflux disease: a systematic review and meta-analysis. Endoscopy. 2018;50(07):708–25.
23. Xie P, Yan J, Ye L, et al. Efficacy of different endoscopic treatments in patients with gastroesophageal reflux disease: a systematic review and network meta-analysis. Surg Endosc. 2021;35(4):1500–10.
24. Haseeb M, Brown JRG, Hayat U, et al. Impact of second-generation transoral incisionless fundoplication on atypical GERD symptoms: a systematic review and meta-analysis. Gastrointest Endosc. 2023;97(3):394–406.e2.
25. Testoni P, Testoni S, Distefano G, et al. Transoral incisionless fundoplication with EsophyX for gastroesophageal reflux disease: clinical efficacy is maintained up to 10 years. Endosc Int Open. 2019;07(05):E647–54.

26. Kim HJ, Kwon CI, Kessler WR, et al. Long-term follow-up results of endoscopic treatment of gastroesophageal reflux disease with the MUSE™ endoscopic stapling device. Surg Endosc. 2016;30(8):3402–8.
27. Zacherl J, Roy-Shapira A, Bonavina L, et al. Endoscopic anterior fundoplication with the Medigus ultrasonic surgical Endostapler (MUSE™) for gastroesophageal reflux disease: 6-month results from a multi-center prospective trial. Surg Endosc. 2015;29(1):220–9.
28. Danalioglu A, Cipe G, Toydemir T, et al. Endoscopic stapling in comparison to laparoscopic fundoplication for the treatment of gastroesophageal reflux disease. Dig Endosc. 2014;26(1):37–42.
29. Yew KC, Chuah SK. Antireflux endoluminal therapies: past and present. Gastroenterol Res Pract. 2013;2013:481417.
30. Pleskow D, Rothstein R, Lo S, et al. Endoscopic full-thickness plication for the treatment of GERD: 12-month follow-up for the north American open-label trial. Gastrointest Endosc. 2005;61(6):643–9.
31. Pleskow D, Rothstein R, Kozarek R, et al. Endoscopic full-thickness plication for the treatment of GERD: five-year long-term multicenter results. Surg Endosc. 2008;22(2):326–32.
32. Weitzendorfer M, Spaun GO, Antoniou SA, et al. Clinical feasibility of a new full-thickness endoscopic plication device (GERDx™) for patients with GERD: results of a prospective trial. Surg Endosc. 2018;32(5):2541–9.
33. Weitzendorfer M, Spaun GO, Antoniou SA, et al. Interim report of a prospective trial on the clinical efficiency of a new full-thickness endoscopic plication device for patients with GERD: impact of changed suture material. Surg Laparosc Endosc Percutan Tech. 2017;27(3):163–9.
34. Kalapala R, Karyampudi A, Nabi Z, et al. Endoscopic full-thickness plication for the treatment of PPI-dependent GERD: results from a randomised, sham controlled trial. Gut. 2022;71(4):686–94.
35. Inoue H, Ito H, Ikeda H, et al. Anti-reflux mucosectomy for gastroesophageal reflux disease in the absence of hiatus hernia: a pilot study. Ann Gastroenterol. 2014;27(4):346–51.
36. Garg R, Mohammed A, Singh A, et al. Anti-reflux mucosectomy for refractory gastroesophageal reflux disease: a systematic review and meta-analysis. Endosc Int Open. 2022;10(06):E854–64.
37. Inoue H, Tanabe M, De Santiago ER, et al. Anti-reflux mucosal ablation (ARMA) as a new treatment for gastroesophageal reflux refractory to proton pump inhibitors: a pilot study. Endosc Int Open. 2020;08(02):E133–8.
38. Shimamura Y, Inoue H, Tanabe M, et al. Clinical outcomes of anti-reflux mucosal ablation for gastroesophageal reflux disease: an international bi-institutional study. J Gastroenterol Hepatol. 2024;39(1):149–56.

Open Access This chapter is licensed under the terms of the Creative Commons Attribution-NonCommercial 4.0 International License (http://creativecommons.org/licenses/by-nc/4.0/), which permits any noncommercial use, sharing, adaptation, distribution and reproduction in any medium or format, as long as you give appropriate credit to the original author(s) and the source, provide a link to the Creative Commons license and indicate if changes were made.

The images or other third party material in this chapter are included in the chapter's Creative Commons license, unless indicated otherwise in a credit line to the material. If material is not included in the chapter's Creative Commons license and your intended use is not permitted by statutory regulation or exceeds the permitted use, you will need to obtain permission directly from the copyright holder.

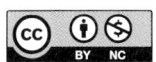

Treatment of Antireflux Surgery Complications

Mario Morino and Elettra Ugliono

15.1 Introduction

Laparoscopic fundoplication is the most commonly performed surgical procedure for the treatment of gastroesophageal reflux disease (GERD). It is highly effective in controlling GERD symptoms, with reported satisfaction rates of 85–90%, even at long-term follow-up.

Nevertheless, despite its success, the literature reports variable failure rates after antireflux surgery, ranging from 3–30%, and surgical revision is required in 3–6% of cases [1]. Despite the lack of consensus, failure is generally defined as the persistence, recurrence, or new onset of adverse gastrointestinal symptoms after antireflux surgery requiring medical attention.

The aim of laparoscopic fundoplication is to restore an efficient antireflux valve in order to prevent the retrograde reflux of gastric content towards the esophagus, without hindering the regular progression of food transit through the esophagogastric junction; obtaining the right balance is not trivial. Furthermore, the esophagogastric junction is an anatomically complex dynamic area subjected to considerable mechanical stress, which can cause herniation or slippage of the fundoplication. The management of failure after fundoplication remains challenging; although published series on redo surgery report satisfactory results in terms of anatomical resolution of the defect, the clinical outcomes are less favorable than with primary surgery. Furthermore, revisional surgery is associated with an increased risk of postoperative morbidity and mortality [2].

Complications after laparoscopic fundoplication can occur both in acute and chronic settings. This chapter focuses on the most commonly reported complications after antireflux surgery, and provides an overview of the diagnostic approach and treatment.

M. Morino (✉) · E. Ugliono
Department of Surgical Sciences, University of Turin, Turin, Italy
e-mail: mario.morino@unito.it; elettra.ugliono@gmail.com

15.2 Acute Complications

Acute complications can occur during the procedure or in the immediate postoperative period, and should be rapidly recognized and addressed to avoid unfortunate sequelae.

Bleeding is the most common complication that can be encountered during laparoscopic fundoplication and, fortunately, is generally minor and easily controlled. Nevertheless, severe bleeding may occur due to an injury of the short gastric vessels or the splenic capsule during gastric fundus mobilization. To prevent this complication, it is essential to avoid excessive traction on the stomach during dissection and perform careful hemostasis in case of division of the short gastric vessels. Furthermore, it is prudent to keep the dissection plane close to the stomach since potential bleeding is easier to control on the gastric side. The better surgical visualization offered by the laparoscopic approach has led to a dramatic reduction in the need for urgent splenectomy, dropping from 4% of the laparotomic series to 0.2–0.5% [3]. In cases of severe uncontrolled bleeding, prompt conversion is strongly recommended.

The reported incidence of visceral perforation during fundoplication is 0–4% and generally involves the esophagus or the stomach [2]. Serosal tearing may result from extensive adhesiolysis or excessive traction on the stomach during gastric mobilization, especially in cases of large hiatal hernias or revisional surgery, where the previous fundoplication may be surrounded by dense adhesions and scar tissue, making the reduction into the abdominal cavity laborious. Perforation is also a particular concern during the passage of the esophageal bougie, which must be performed by experienced operators, and during the construction of a stapled Collis gastroplasty. If in doubt of a perforation, an air-leak test should be performed to assess the integrity of the esophageal and gastric walls. While a gastric perforation can be safely managed by laparoscopic suturing, esophageal lesions are challenging to repair both by laparoscopy or laparotomy.

Pleural injury can occur when dissection is performed in the mediastinum, especially in complex situations such as the presence of a large hiatal hernia, short esophagus, or during revisional surgery, where it is reported in up to 10% of cases [4]. Opening the pleura allows carbon dioxide to flow into the pleural space causing pneumothorax, leading to increased air pressures, hypotension, and loss of vision in the surgical field. When recognized, it should be promptly addressed by draining the pleural cavity: a small cannula inserted during the procedure allows resolution of the pneumothorax, while repair by suturing is not always needed.

15.3 Chronic Complications

The long-term persistence of symptoms, or the appearance of severe symptoms, requires the performance of diagnostic tests. Chronic complications can be divided into functional and structural complications, if anatomical abnormalities are documented at instrumental examinations.

15.4 Functional Complications

15.4.1 Dysphagia

Mild dysphagia is commonly observed in the immediate postoperative period after antireflux surgery, occurring in approximately 70% of patients. This condition, caused by the inflammation and post-surgical edema of the wrap, is generally mild and transient, resolving spontaneously within 2–3 months. However, 3–24% of patients experience persistent dysphagia, requiring further instrumental investigations [5]. Upper gastrointestinal endoscopy and radiological contrast studies are recommended to exclude the presence of structural complications. Furthermore, endoscopic biopsy samples at the proximal and distal esophagus are helpful to rule out a preoperatively undiagnosed eosinophilic esophagitis.

In the absence of structural complications, some degree of dysphagia, particularly for solid foods, is considered a plausible regular sequela of laparoscopic fundoplication. This artificial wrap, in fact, does not possess some of the intrinsic functional characteristics of the native lower esophageal sphincter, such as the ability to open in a coordinated manner with the arrival of the peristalsis wave at the level of the distal esophagus and the ability to guarantee transient relaxations of the lower esophageal sphincter.

These symptoms can be exacerbated in the presence of esophageal motor disorders, such as ineffective esophageal motility. In order to reduce the incidence of postoperative dysphagia, some authors have proposed a "tailored" approach to fundoplication depending on the peristaltic characteristics of the patient. The hypothesis underlying this concept is that partial fundoplication, causing a reduced obstructive effect at the level of the esophagogastric junction, leads to a lower degree of dysphagia in patients with insufficient peristaltic reserve. This approach has long been debated, and several clinical studies have demonstrated that esophageal motility does not influence surgical outcomes.

Several studies have been conducted but have failed to identify predictors of postoperative dysphagia; recently, provocative high-resolution esophageal manometry maneuvers appear to be reliable in assessing peristaltic reserve and may have a role in identifying patients at higher risk for postoperative dysphagia.

15.4.2 Gastroesophageal Reflux Disease Recurrence

Persistent or recurrent GERD-like symptoms are occasionally reported after laparoscopic fundoplication and can be ascribed to several clinical situations requiring a stepwise analysis. First of all, the presence of structural complications, eventually requiring revisional surgery, should be excluded. Persistent GERD symptoms immediately after surgery can be due to a structural laxity of the fundoplication caused by technical errors in the construction of the wrap. Recurrence of GERD after initial satisfactory outcomes can be subsequent to wrap destruction, resulting in the failure of the procedure.

If no structural complications are identified by means of endoscopy and X-ray barium meal, recurrent reflux may be due to the declining effectiveness of fundoplication over time. Although published studies report excellent functional results that are maintained even at 20 years of follow-up, the precise durability of the effects of fundoplication is not known.

However, symptoms alone are not enough to diagnose GERD recurrence, and objective evidence of pathologic reflux is mandatory. In fact, according to data from long-term randomized controlled trials comparing antireflux surgery and medical therapy, abnormal pH monitoring occurred in approximately 20% of patients who reported recurrent GERD symptoms after fundoplication [5, 6].

Over time, resumption of antiacid medications occurs in approximately one-third of patients; however, proton-pump inhibitors are often given empirically without prior objective documentation of reflux, and other causes may justify their prescription, such as peptic ulcer disease or concomitant use of gastro-toxic drugs.

When persistent or recurrent GERD is suspected, pHmetric monitoring is helpful in objectively documenting the presence and severity of reflux, and establishing the relationship between reflux episodes and symptoms, since recurrent symptoms may not depend on reflux, in order to optimize the medical management.

15.4.3 Gas-Bloat Syndrome

Gas-bloat syndrome is a clinical condition characterized by abdominal distension, early satiety, nausea, flatulence, and abdominal pain. The etiopathogenesis is not clearly defined, but it is presumed to depend on the inability, after fundoplication, to vent air from the stomach in response to gastric distension, an event that commonly occurs with belching. Due to the lack of a precise definition of this clinical condition, the incidence of gas-bloat syndrome after fundoplication is highly variable, ranging between 1% and 85%. These symptoms appear to be more severe after total than after partial fundoplication, and are exacerbated in the case of delayed gastric emptying [7]. Treatment of gas-bloat syndrome is conservative and consists of avoiding fermented foods and carbonated drinks, reducing aerophagia during meals, smoking cessation, gas-reducing drugs, and prokinetics.

In cases of severe and persistent symptoms, instrumental examinations are indicated to exclude other etiologies, such as intestinal subocclusion and gastroparesis due to vagal lesions. Surgical reintervention may be considered only in the case of debilitating symptoms. Possible strategies include take-down of the fundoplication, conversion of total to partial fundoplication, and partial gastrectomy; however, there is no evidence in the literature reporting the effectiveness of these procedures in resolving symptoms.

15.5 Structural Complications

Structural complications after antireflux surgery are reported in up to 30% of cases, and manifest clinically with persistent dysphagia or recurrent reflux.

15.5.1 Technical Operative Principles

It is necessary to pay attention to compliance with some technical principles to ensure a correctly constructed fundoplication. The esophagus must be adequately mobilized, possibly proceeding with an extended mediastinal dissection, in order to obtain at least 3 cm of intra-abdominal esophageal length without tension. Similarly, adequate gastric fundus mobilization should be verified by performing the "shoeshine" maneuver: the surgeon grasps the medial and lateral edges of the wrap and pulls them back and forth behind the esophagus to assess the absence of tension and to check that the correct portion of the stomach is used for the construction of the fundoplication, without twisting. The fundoplication must be positioned precisely over the esophagogastric junction, rather than the stomach. Finally, a properly built total fundoplication should follow the criteria described by DeMeester; therefore, it should be short (approximately 2 cm long) and floppy [8]. An esophageal bougie could be used to prevent excessively tight wraps. In cases of large hiatal hernia the closure of the diaphragm could be challenging: a posterior interrupted suture using non-resorbable material and loosely calibrated on the esophagus constitutes the technique of choice. In the case of weakened diaphragmatic pillars or a large diaphragmatic opening, reinforcement of the hiatus with prosthetic materials can be performed. The cruroplasty must always be performed posteriorly to the esophagus, to avoid excessive angulation.

15.5.2 Diagnosis of Structural Complications

Upper gastrointestinal endoscopy and contrast-medium radiological series are the primary diagnostic modalities for evaluating structural complications after fundoplication.

Endoscopy allows the evaluation of the integrity of the esophageal mucosa and the detection of esophagitis, a possible expression of recurrent GERD. The presence of stenosis at the esophagogastric junction can be evaluated by findings of food stagnation in the esophagus and by the difficulty in the passage of the scope at the cardia level. Furthermore, it is possible to assess the location, orientation, and integrity of the antireflux valve, and its relationship with the diaphragm; the fundoplication should be located just below the diaphragmatic impression. The presence of the wrap above the diaphragmatic impression indicates the herniation of the fundoplication into the chest.

A contrast-medium radiological series provides additional information on the extraluminal anatomy of the esophagogastric junction, the exact location of the fundoplication, the length of the esophagus, and the presence of a possible paraesophageal component.

15.5.3 Classification

Horgan et al. published an excellent anatomic classification of structural complications, based on the preoperative work-up and operative findings after revisional surgery [9] (Fig. 15.1).

Type I: herniation of the wrap through the esophagogastric junction

- Type Ia: herniation involving fundoplication
- Type Ib: herniation not involving fundoplication.

Type II: herniation of a paraesophageal component resulting in a redundant fundoplication.

Type III: malformation (localization or construction defect) of the fundoplication. These anomalies include defects in the creation of the fundoplication (too wide or too narrow), excessive closure of the hiatal defect, excessive angulation.

Type Ia is the most common structural complication, reported in 30–80% of cases [4]. This type of failure results from a disrupted cruroplasty or failure to obtain adequate esophageal mobilization during the dissection phase of the procedure. Several technical elements are fundamental to reducing the risk of developing this complication. The esophagus should be dissected to obtain at least 3 cm of intra-abdominal esophageal length. Lengthening procedures, such as Collis gastroplasty, should be considered if a short esophagus is detected intraoperatively and a sufficient esophageal length cannot be achieved despite extensive mediastinal dissection. Furthermore, cruroplasty must be free of tension; in the case of weakened diaphragmatic pillars or a large diaphragmatic opening that does not allow complete closure of the defect, cruroplasty with mesh can be performed. Intraoperative endoscopy could be useful to evaluate the extent of the esophageal mobilization [10].

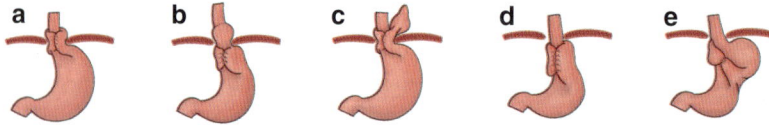

Fig. 15.1 Classification of structural complications. (Adapted from Horgan et al. [9]). (**a**) Type Ia: herniation through the esophagogastric junction involving the fundoplication. (**b**) Type Ib: herniation through the esophagogastric junction not involving the fundoplication. (**c**) Type II: herniation of a paraesophageal component. (**d**) Type III: malformation of the fundoplication (excessively long fundoplication). (**e**) Type III: malformation of the fundoplication (bicompartmental stomach)

Type Ib is the so-called slipped fundoplication, reported in 15–30% of cases. It occurs when a portion of the stomach below the fundoplication migrates through it, and herniates above the diaphragm, leaving the fundoplication in the correct position. The leading cause of slipping is a structural laxity of the fundoplication or an incorrect wrap construction at the time of the first operation. To avoid this complication, attention must be paid to choosing the correct part of the stomach that will be used to perform the fundoplication, assessed with the "shoe-shine" maneuver. The insertion of an esophageal bougie could be helpful for the calibration of the wrap at the correct tension.

Type II failure consists of a paraesophageal hernia. The mechanism underlying the onset of this complication is associated with a poorly constructed fundoplication with excessive redundant gastric tissue and associated ineffective hiatal closure. The herniated gastric portion causes external compression at the esophagogastric junction, resulting in persistent dysphagia. As for type II failure, this complication is prevented by the performance of the "shoe-shine" maneuver.

Type III failures constitute 10% of structural complications. They result from other errors in the construction of the fundoplication, such as a fundoplication that is too tight or too long or a bicompartmental stomach that causes a stenosis at the level of the cardia. A tight fundoplication is a fundoplication that does not meet the DeMeester "short and floppy" criteria to avoid postoperative dysphagia. The construction of the fundoplication with the help of an esophageal bougie could reduce these complications. Furthermore, dysphagia secondary to tight fundoplication can improve with postoperative endoscopic dilations in the majority of cases [7].

15.5.4 Revisional Surgery

Surgical revision should be considered in patients with evidence of structural abnormalities and severely debilitating symptoms that are not controlled by medical or endoscopic therapy. Overall, approximately 3–5% of patients will require redo surgery [2].

Revisional surgery is technically demanding and is associated with higher morbidity and mortality. Functional outcomes are often worse than the primary procedure and may not meet patient expectations [11].

Several technical steps must be accomplished when approaching revisional surgery after fundoplication; regardless of the cause of failure and the indication for surgery, the first step of the procedure must be the restoration of normal anatomy, achieved through the complete take-down of the previous fundoplication and restoration of the gastric fundus to its normal position.

Once normal gastric anatomy is achieved, the hiatus and the esophagus must be carefully examined to better identify the cause of the failure. The esophagus should be fully mobilized and checked for the presence of a short esophagus [10]. Lengthening procedures, such as Collis gastroplasty, should be performed if sufficient esophageal intra-abdominal length without tension is not achieved. During these maneuvers, care must be taken to preserve the vagal nerves.

If a hiatal hernia recurrence occurs, it must be gently reduced in the abdomen and the crural defect closed. If the sutures are not likely to hold due to excessive tension or weak pillars, crural repair can be reinforced with mesh.

There is currently no consensus on the best reoperative strategy for patients requiring revisional surgery after laparoscopic fundoplication. Possible surgical strategies include, depending on the specific cause of failure, construction of a loose Nissen fundoplication over an esophageal bougie or conversion to partial posterior fundoplication; another reasonable alternative is the conversion to a Roux-en-Y gastric bypass, especially for patients with higher body mass index values, patients with severe esophageal dysmotility and with suspected vagal nerve injury [12].

References

1. Dallemagne B, Arenas Sanchez M, Francart D, et al. Long-term results after laparoscopic reoperation for failed antireflux procedures. Br J Surg. 2011;98:1581–7.
2. Stefanidis D, Hope WW, Kohn GP, et al. Guidelines for surgical treatment of gastroesophageal reflux disease. Surg Endosc. 2010;24:2647–69.
3. Bizekis C, Kent M, Luketich J. Complications after surgery for gastroesophageal reflux disease. Thorac Surg Clin. 2006;16:99–108.
4. Richter JE. Gastroesophageal reflux disease treatment: side effects and complications of fundoplication. Clin Gastroenterol Hepatol. 2013;11:465–71. quiz e39
5. Lundell L, Attwood S, Ell C, et al. Comparing laparoscopic antireflux surgery with esomeprazole in the management of patients with chronic gastro-oesophageal reflux disease: a 3-year interim analysis of the LOTUS trial. Gut. 2008;57:1207–13.
6. Grant AM, Boachie C, Cotton SC, et al. Clinical and economic evaluation of laparoscopic surgery compared with medical management for gastro-oesophageal reflux disease: 5-year follow-up of multicentre randomised trial (the REFLUX trial). Health Technol Assess. 2013;17:1–167.
7. Sobrino-Cossío S, Soto-Pérez JC, Coss-Adame E, et al. Post-fundoplication symptoms and complications: diagnostic approach and treatment. Rev Gastroenterol Mex. 2017;82:234–47.
8. DeMeester TR, Bonavina L, Albertucci M. Nissen fundoplication for gastroesophageal reflux disease. Evaluation of primary repair in 100 consecutive patients. Ann Surg. 1986;204:9–20.
9. Horgan S, Pellegrini CA. Surgical treatment of gastroesophageal reflux disease. Surg Clin North Am. 1997;77:1063–82.
10. Mattioli S, Lugaresi ML, Costantini M, et al. The short esophagus: intraoperative assessment of esophageal length. J Thorac Cardiovasc Surg. 2008;136:834–41.
11. Yadlapati R, Vaezi MF, Vela MF, et al. Management options for patients with GERD and persistent symptoms on proton pump inhibitors: recommendations from an expert panel. Am J Gastroenterol. 2018;113:980–6.
12. Shao JM, Elhage SA, Prasad T, et al. Best reoperative strategy for failed fundoplication: redo fundoplication or conversion to roux-en-Y gastric diversion? Surg Endosc. 2021;35:3865–73.

15 Treatment of Antireflux Surgery Complications

Open Access This chapter is licensed under the terms of the Creative Commons Attribution-NonCommercial 4.0 International License (http://creativecommons.org/licenses/by-nc/4.0/), which permits any noncommercial use, sharing, adaptation, distribution and reproduction in any medium or format, as long as you give appropriate credit to the original author(s) and the source, provide a link to the Creative Commons license and indicate if changes were made.

The images or other third party material in this chapter are included in the chapter's Creative Commons license, unless indicated otherwise in a credit line to the material. If material is not included in the chapter's Creative Commons license and your intended use is not permitted by statutory regulation or exceeds the permitted use, you will need to obtain permission directly from the copyright holder.

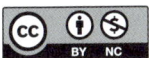

Obesity, Bariatric Surgery and Gastroesophageal Reflux Disease

16

Salvatore Tolone and Ludovico Docimo

16.1 Introduction, Context, and Diagnosis of GERD in Obese Patients

Obesity today is one of the most prevalent chronic diseases worldwide, representing a genuine global health crisis, aptly referred to as "globesity". Beyond its impact on quality of life, obesity significantly raises the risk of numerous comorbidities, including type II diabetes, cardiovascular disease, and certain cancers. The gastrointestinal system is particularly affected, with obesity linked to gallstones, the progression of fatty liver diseases like non-alcoholic steatohepatitis and non-alcoholic fatty liver disease to cirrhosis, and increased risk of colorectal conditions such as diverticulitis, polyps, and colorectal cancer [1].

Notably, obesity doubles the risk of gastroesophageal reflux disease (GERD), erosive esophagitis, and quadruples the likelihood of Barrett's esophagus, alongside heightened risks for esophageal and gastric adenocarcinomas (Table 16.1). Thus, obesity is an independent risk factor for developing GERD, esophagitis, and hiatal hernia. A study on 1659 patients revealed that as body mass index (BMI) increases, lower esophageal sphincter (LES) pressure decreases, raising the incidence of erosive esophagitis. Central obesity is associated with increased exposure to acid reflux in the distal esophagus, a shorter LES, and extended cardial mucosa, which produces additional acid just below the LES. Even asymptomatic obese patients show elevated intra-esophageal acid exposure and more frequent reflux episodes in pH testing compared to normal-weight individuals.

This phenomenon is partly due to increased waist circumference, central fat, and intra-abdominal pressure, which heighten the risk of disrupting the normal anatomical barrier at the gastroesophageal junction, often leading to hiatal hernia.

S. Tolone (✉) · L. Docimo
UOC General, Mininvasive, Oncological and Bariatric Surgery,
University of Campania "Luigi Vanvitelli", Naples, Italy
e-mail: salvatore.tolone@unicampania.it; ludovico.docimo@unicampania.it

Table 16.1 Proposed mechanisms for gastroesophageal reflux disease (GERD) development in obese patients

Increased intra-abdominal pressure	Higher frequency of hiatal hernia (sliding type)	More frequent LES hypotonia	Increased number of TLESRs
Larger meal portions	Greater intake of foods and beverages affecting acidity and LES tone	Reduced esophageal mucosal sensitivity to acid	Increased minor motility disorders, especially IEM
Impact of central adiposity on gastrointestinal hormones			

IEM ineffective esophageal motility, *LES* lower esophageal sphincter, *TLESRs* transient lower esophageal sphincter relaxations

Additionally, factors like adiponectin, leptin, and high-fat, high-calorie foods further exacerbate LES hypotension or cause temporary involuntary relaxations.

The correlation between obesity and increased GERD symptoms and esophagitis is clear, as effective weight loss reduces GERD symptoms, proton-pump inhibitor (PPI) use, and mucosal injury. The gastroesophageal junction, a complex anatomical zone, must maintain integrity to prevent reflux; obesity undermines this, complicating GERD management in obese patients.

Obese patients may exhibit silent GERD, lacking typical symptoms despite high acid exposure, suggesting that diagnosing GERD purely based on symptoms may be inadequate in this population. Research suggests the Montreal Consensus definition of GERD is reliable for only a third of obese patients. "Silent reflux" may contribute to higher rates of symptomatic GERD after bariatric surgery. Therefore, the diagnostic algorithm from the Lyon Consensus 2.0 is crucial for accurate GERD diagnosis in obese patients. Instrumental tests are essential to document and confirm GERD presence and verify symptom-reflux correlations [2–4].

While the Lyon Consensus 2.0 provides a structured diagnostic approach, it is based on data from non-obese populations. However, high-resolution esophageal manometry (HRM) and pH monitoring remain gold standards for GERD assessment in obese patients. HRM is especially valuable before bariatric surgery, assessing the esophagogastric junction (EGJ) morphology and separating the LES from the diaphragmatic crura, essential for identifying and confirming hiatal hernias and evaluating EGJ function. HRM demonstrated 90% sensitivity and at least 65% specificity for hiatal hernia detection, surpassing endoscopy and radiology, even in obese candidates for bariatric surgery.

HRM's high accuracy in confirming type III EGJ hernias (over 3 cm) is clinically relevant, with abnormal pH monitoring in over 95% of these cases. Therefore, hiatal hernia assessment in obese patients, especially those undergoing bariatric surgery, is critical. Furthermore, pH impedance testing, which evaluates weakly acidic and weakly alkaline reflux, is vital for obese "volume eaters" or "nibblers", who may experience post-meal reflux that is partially buffered by food.

Current GERD diagnostic protocols in obese patients align with the Lyon Consensus 2.0 guidelines, but normative values for HRM, pH monitoring, and endoscopy are primarily based on non-obese populations. Only one existing study provides normative HRM data in asymptomatic obese individuals, and broader research is needed for a global consensus [5].

16.2 Effects of Bariatric Surgery on GERD

16.2.1 Why Is Reflux Assessment Crucial for Obese Patients?

Numerous case series have documented esophageal functional studies conducted prior to bariatric surgery, which reveal that at least 30% of asymptomatic obese patients may have esophageal dysmotility (commonly ineffective peristalsis, followed by distal esophageal spasm [DES], or esophagogastric junction outflow obstruction [EGJ-OO]) or positive reflux monitoring. Given these findings, researchers have questioned whether the presence of pathological or borderline gastroesophageal reflux, symptomatic or not, could lead to long-term consequences following different bariatric procedures.

The most widely performed bariatric procedure globally, sleeve gastrectomy, involves a vertical or "sleeved" resection of the stomach. Sleeve gastrectomy has generated significant debate in recent years due to evidence suggesting that it may contribute to chronic, medication-resistant GERD. Observational trials have shown that over 30% of patients develop reflux esophagitis following this procedure, with Barrett's esophagus appearing in up to 17% of cases. However, studies involving strict patient selection—excluding those with hiatal hernias, esophageal dysmotility, or pathological acid exposure—demonstrated no *de novo* GERD after sleeve gastrectomy, indicating that this procedure is safe for well-assessed obese patients [6].

The mechanisms behind the reflux-promoting potential of sleeve gastrectomy are documented in various studies. Risk factors for developing or worsening GERD after the procedure include undiagnosed GERD, uncorrected hiatal hernia, stomach resection close to the angle of His (compromising LES muscle fibers), excessive resection of the antrum (leading to bile reflux from the loss of the antral pump), and mid-gastric stenosis. The resection of the gastric fundus in sleeve gastrectomy reduces the stomach's ability to maintain isobaric conditions, causing increased intragastric pressure even after small meals and resulting in postprandial reflux (Table 16.2).

16.2.2 Adjustable Gastric Banding and GERD

Another restrictive bariatric technique, adjustable gastric banding, also has a potential for inducing reflux and esophageal dysmotility, including pseudoachalasia. This procedure restricts food passage through a narrowing created just below the

Table 16.2 Proposed pathophysiological mechanisms for the development or worsening of gastroesophageal reflux disease (GERD) or dysmotility following common bariatric surgery procedures

Bariatric surgery procedure	Proposed mechanisms
Sleeve gastrectomy	Intragastric hyperpressure, cutting of LES fibers leading to hypotonia, mid-gastric stenosis, excessive antral resection, untreated hiatal hernia, silent preoperative GERD, intrathoracic migration of the sleeve, excessive fundus resection, induction of ineffective peristalsis.
Gastric banding	Hourglass-like transit effect, induced LES hypotonia, overtightened band, band mispositioned over LES, creation of EGJ-OO, induction of pseudo-achalasia.
Single anastomosis gastric bypass	Short gastric pouch, excessively wide gastric pouch, short biliary limb, difficult transit through gastrojejunal anastomosis, untreated hiatal hernia, LES hypotonia.
Roux-en-Y gastric bypass	LES hypotonia, challenging transit through gastrojejunal anastomosis, short biliary limb, candy cane syndrome, untreated hiatal hernia.

EGJ-OO esophagogastric junction outflow obstruction, *LES* lower esophageal sphincter

gastroesophageal junction, which can inadvertently recreate the reflux mechanism seen with hiatal hernias. If the band shifts upwards or tightens, it can obstruct the gastroesophageal junction, causing dysphagia and esophageal dilation, identified on HRM as hypercontractile motility patterns or EGJ-OO. Severe cases resemble pseudoachalasia, stemming from external obstruction rather than a primary motility disorder.

16.2.3 Roux-en-Y Gastric Bypass

Data on other popular procedures, such as Roux-en-Y gastric bypass (RYGB), are mixed. Traditionally, RYGB has been viewed as an effective antireflux procedure in obese patients with GERD, often recommended as the first-line treatment for obese individuals with GERD and a BMI over 30 or 35. Although many studies support RYGB's ability to control GERD through weight loss, reduced gastric pouch capacity, and creation of a low-pressure "common cavity" at the gastrojejunostomy, recent research indicates that long-term control may be symptomatic rather than physiological. Nearly 50% of RYGB patients report ongoing GERD symptoms or exhibit abnormal pH monitoring results over time, particularly if hiatal hernia repair was omitted, the gastrojejunostomy is slow to empty, or the LES is hypotonic.

Given these findings, the effectiveness of RYGB in GERD control may depend on addressing key antireflux surgery principles, such as hiatal hernia repair and restoring LES pressure, although LES reconstruction is challenging without a fundoplication (which, if added to RYGB, lacks functionality due to the inactive remnant stomach). Furthermore, RYGB bypasses the duodenum, impairing the absorption of PPIs; therefore, open-capsule or dispersible PPIs may be preferable for these patients.

16.2.4 Single Anastomosis Gastric Bypass

Single anastomosis gastric bypass (SAGB) also shows potential as a GERD management strategy, although some studies associate it with a physiology similar to the Billroth II procedure. Research on patients without preoperative hiatal hernia or GERD shows that SAGB can even reduce reflux as measured by pH-impedance, with negligible weakly alkaline reflux. Some researchers attribute this effect to the weight loss and elevated intragastric pressure generated by the gastric pouch, which, similar to sleeve gastrectomy, allows bile to flow into the alimentary loop without refluxing. However, if the pouch is too short or wide, or the biliary limb too short, bile stasis and bile reflux may occur. Converting SAGB to RYGB is recommended in such cases [7–9].

16.2.5 Emerging Variants and Future Directions

New sleeve gastrectomy variants that incorporate fundoplication aim to control reflux without altering the gastrointestinal anatomy. Fundoplication types like Dor, Toupet, Nissen, and Nissen-Rossetti paired with sleeve gastrectomy have shown promising results in small, single-center studies, reducing *de novo* or worsening reflux. However, further research is needed to confirm these findings.

Ultimately, obesity presents a significant risk to the functional integrity of the gastroesophageal junction, with many obese patients experiencing asymptomatic reflux. Since some bariatric procedures may exacerbate or induce GERD, comprehensive preoperative evaluation following established GERD diagnostic protocols is essential. Knowledge of the mechanisms behind reflux after these surgeries and modifications to traditional techniques, such as adding fundoplication to sleeve gastrectomy, could minimize reflux-related risks as these approaches are further researched and potentially integrated into clinical practice.

References

1. De Luca M, Shikora S, Eisenberg D, et al. Scientific evidence for the updated guidelines on indications for metabolic and bariatric surgery (IFSO/ASMBS). Obes Surg. 2024;34(11):3963–4096.
2. Pandolfino JE, El-Serag HB, Zhang Q, et al. Obesity: a challenge to esophagogastric junction integrity. Gastroenterology. 2006;130(3):639–49.
3. El-Serag HB, Ergun GA, Pandolfino J, et al. Obesity increases oesophageal acid exposure. Gut. 2007;56(6):749–55.
4. Ayazi S, Hagen JA, Chan LS, et al. Obesity and gastroesophageal reflux: quantifying the association between body mass index, esophageal acid exposure, and lower esophageal sphincter status in a large series of patients with reflux symptoms. J Gastrointest Surg. 2009;13(8):1440–7.
5. Yadlapati R, Gyawali CP, Pandolfino JE. CGIT GERD consensus conference participants. AGA clinical practice update on the personalized approach to the evaluation and management of GERD: expert review. Clin Gastroenterol Hepatol. 2022;20(5):984–994.e1.
6. Sebastianelli L, Benois M, Vanbiervliet G, et al. Systematic endoscopy 5 years after sleeve gastrectomy results in a high rate of Barrett's esophagus: results of a multicenter study. Obes Surg. 2019;29(5):1462–9.

7. Tolone S, Conzo G, Flagiello L, et al. De novo gastroesophageal reflux disease symptoms are infrequent after sleeve gastrectomy at 2-year follow-up using a comprehensive preoperative esophageal assessment. J Clin Med. 2024;13(2):545.
8. Tolone S, Savarino E, de Bortoli N, et al. Esophageal high-resolution manometry can unravel the mechanisms by which different bariatric techniques produce different reflux exposures. J Gastrointest Surg. 2020;24(1):1–7.
9. Loo JH, Chue KM, Lim CH, et al. Effectiveness of sleeve gastrectomy plus fundoplication versus sleeve gastrectomy alone for treatment of patients with severe obesity: a systematic review and meta-analysis. Surg Obes Relat Dis. 2024;20(6):532–43.

Open Access This chapter is licensed under the terms of the Creative Commons Attribution-NonCommercial 4.0 International License (http://creativecommons.org/licenses/by-nc/4.0/), which permits any noncommercial use, sharing, adaptation, distribution and reproduction in any medium or format, as long as you give appropriate credit to the original author(s) and the source, provide a link to the Creative Commons license and indicate if changes were made.

The images or other third party material in this chapter are included in the chapter's Creative Commons license, unless indicated otherwise in a credit line to the material. If material is not included in the chapter's Creative Commons license and your intended use is not permitted by statutory regulation or exceeds the permitted use, you will need to obtain permission directly from the copyright holder.

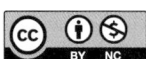

Clinical Evaluation, Etiology and Classification of Esophageal Achalasia

17

Mario Costantini and Andrea Costantini

17.1 Definition and Epidemiology

Although rare, achalasia is the most frequent primary esophageal motility disorder, with a reported incidence of about 0.5–1 new case in 100,000 adult individuals a year, and only 0.18/100,000/year in the pediatric population [1]. It is usually diagnosed between 20 and 50 years of age, but it can occur at any age, including age extremes, with no difference between male and female subjects [1]. It was first described (and treated) by Sir Thomas Willis in 1674, who referred to it as "cardiospasm". This concept held the field until 1915, when Hertz [2] suggested that the disease was a syndrome caused by the failure of the cardia to relax on swallowing. He named the condition *achalasia*, from the Greek verb meaning "failure to relax" (α- privative = not; $\chi\alpha\lambda\acute{\alpha}\omega$ = I relax).

Left untreated, achalasia frequently progresses towards a dilation of the esophagus, which gradually becomes increasingly enlarged until it acquires an end-stage sigmoid shape, with retention of liquids, saliva and undigested food. The most common form of achalasia is idiopathic achalasia, mostly occurring as sporadic cases. However, a similar clinical presentation can be seen in patients with Chagas disease, caused by infection with *Trypanosoma cruzi*, or even with the so-called "pseudoachalasia", characterized by degeneration of the myenteric plexus due to neoplastic infiltration by different tumors [1]. Rarely, achalasia can also be part of other

---

M. Costantini (✉)
Department of Surgical, Oncological and Gastroenterological Sciences,
University of Padua, Padua, Italy
e-mail: m.costantini@unipd.it

A. Costantini
Department of Surgical, Oncological and Gastroenterological Sciences,
School of General Surgery, University of Padua, Padua, Italy
e-mail: andrycostantini91@gmail.com

complex syndromes such as the Allgrove syndrome (triple A syndrome: i.e., alacrimia, achalasia and adrenal insufficiency), autism or Down's syndrome [1]. Some familial cases of achalasia have also been described [3]. In this chapter we will limit our discussion to the most common, idiopathic form of the disease.

17.2 Etiology and Pathophysiology

The etiology of achalasia is still unknown, so that any current therapy—by means of endoscopic balloon dilations or surgical or endoscopic myotomy—is palliative and aimed at disrupting the unrelaxing sphincter. What is known so far is that the end result of any causative mechanism is inflammation (ganglionitis) and the subsequent disappearance of the myenteric neurons that coordinate esophageal peristalsis and lower esophageal sphincter (LES) relaxation [1]. Esophageal peristaltic propagation and LES relaxation depend on a well-balanced equilibrium between excitatory (cholinergic) and inhibitory neurons. The latter, mainly using vasoactive intestinal peptide and nitric oxide as transmitters, were found to be reduced or absent in LES specimens from patients with achalasia [4]. Other studies showed infiltration of cytotoxic lymphocytes within the myenteric ganglia; antibodies against myenteric neurons have been shown in serum samples of patients with achalasia [1]. These findings suggest the involvement of an aberrant immune response to antigens which are still unknown. Some viruses, such as herpes simplex virus 1 (HSV-1) [5], measles, and papillomavirus have been proposed as potential antigens [1]. Recently, SARS-CoV2 and its receptor were found in the LES muscle of achalasia patients with COVID-19, but not in controls, suggesting that also coronaviruses may affect the myenteric plexus [6]. HSV-1 DNA has been identified in the esophageal tissue as well, and isolated esophageal T cells from achalasia patients specifically proliferate and release cytokines on exposure to HSV-1 antigens [5]. However, HSV-1 DNA was also identified in the esophagus of control individuals, suggesting that HSV-1 may only trigger an immune activation (and subsequent loss of enteric neurons) in genetically predisposed patients. In fact, an association has been reported between achalasia and gene polymorphisms in HLA class II molecules [1]. Moreover, the rarely described cases of familial achalasia further support a role for genetic factors in the etiopathogenesis of achalasia. In summary, in genetically predisposed subjects, external insults (viruses, toxins) may trigger an aberrant auto-immune response, leading to ganglionitis and progressive loss of myenteric neurons, causing achalasia.

17.3 Clinical Evaluation

The most frequently occurring symptoms of achalasia are dysphagia for solids and liquids (>90%), regurgitation of undigested food (76–91%), chest pain (25–64%), and weight loss (35–91%) [1]. The severity of these symptoms is usually graded with several scoring scales, the Eckardt score being the most widely used [7] despite major criticisms by some authors. This score combines the severity and frequency of dysphagia, regurgitation and pain (0 = never, 1 = occasionally, 2 = daily, 3 = with each meal) with a symptom score of 0–3 for the degree of weight loss, resulting in a maximum overall score of 12. A value of 3 or below is considered normal and reflects the efficacy of the treatment. Dysphagia is capricious and slowly progressive; it may be more severe for liquids than for solids, and it is often aggravated by stressful situations. Chest pain may be reported in all subtypes of achalasia, but particularly in type 3 (see below), and it responds less well to treatment than do dysphagia and regurgitation, which probably explains the less favorable therapeutic results obtained in patients with type 3 achalasia [8]. The exact mechanism underlying chest pain remains unclear but could include the stimulation of chemoreceptors for the acid fermentation of food retained in the esophagus, mucosal inflammation related to stasis, spastic or uncoordinated smooth muscle contractions, esophageal ischemia and/or a lowered esophageal sensitivity threshold [4]. Respiratory complications (nocturnal cough and aspiration) can also be present, especially in patients with substantial stasis of large amounts of food and secretions. Heartburn can be reported in up to 75% of achalasia patients [9]. In these patients, heartburn might result from mechanisms other than classical gastroesophageal reflux disease (GERD): again, both the disordered esophageal motor activity causing spasm and distention of the esophageal wall and the intraluminal acidification resulting from retained food fermentation might produce sensations indistinguishable from heartburn of acid reflux. All this can lead to an erroneous diagnosis of GERD, which might culminate in erroneous antireflux surgery [10]. It must be said, however, that the symptoms of achalasia are not specific, which explains the long delay between the onset of symptoms and the final diagnosis (up to 5 years in some studies) [11]. Patients are often misdiagnosed as cases of heart disease or GERD. They are also often referred to a psychiatrist for suspected eating disorders, especially if they are young women [12].

17.4 Diagnosis

Dysphagia, the principal symptom in achalasia, is the signature symptom of the esophagus, being present virtually in any esophageal disease. It is also an ominous symptom, becoming evident only when a possible neoplastic disease is well advanced. Any patient complaining of difficulty in swallowing must therefore undergo specific tests to obtain a correct diagnosis.

17.5 Upper Endoscopy

Upper endoscopy (with esophageal biopsies) is mandatory to exclude other causes of dysphagia, such as eosinophilic esophagitis, strictures, webs or rings, and above all malignancy, causing "pseudoachalasia", present in 2 to 4% of suspected achalasia cases [1]. Although mandatory, endoscopy is not very sensitive in confirming a diagnosis of achalasia, since more than 40% of patients may have normal endoscopic findings [4]. Indicative for achalasia is the presence of a dilated or tortuous esophagus with saliva and/or food retention, and a tight esophagogastric junction (EGJ) that allows sudden passage of the scope gently pushed by the operator [4]. The presence of esophageal candidiasis refractory to treatment is also common, and related to esophageal stasis: the finding of esophageal candidiasis in patients with an intact immune function should prompt to suspect achalasia or other esophageal motor disorders as the cause of symptoms [4]. Long-standing esophageal stasis may lead to the finding of some form of esophagitis, hence the name "stasis esophagitis", often mistaken for the more common reflux esophagitis and leading to inappropriate treatment with proton-pump inhibitors or, worse, antireflux surgery. If endoscopy is normal, however, a patient complaining of dysphagia must not be dismissed as "functional", and further investigations must be planned to avoid a diagnostic delay or misdiagnosis.

17.6 Barium Swallow

The barium swallow (BS) is an easy-to-perform, inexpensive, and readily repeatable test. However, today it may be difficult to obtain it in a general radiological service not really devoted to esophagus studies. The test specifically aims at assessing the emptying capability and morphology of the esophagus. Its diagnostic sensitivity for diagnosing achalasia is, however, only 60% [13] and there are currently no data about its specificity. BS may show a tapered cardias with the classic "bird's beak" appearance, and a slow passage of the bolus through it. Some dilation of the esophageal body with a barium column in the esophagus with an air-fluid level is pathognomonic for the disease [1]. The absence of an air bubble in the stomach is also a common finding and this should strongly suggest a diagnosis of achalasia [14]. BS also allows disease severity to be graded by classifying patients based on esophageal diameter and shape [15, 16]. In stage I, a slight dilation of the esophagus is observed (<4 cm); in stage II the dilatation is moderate (4–6 cm); and in stage III it is diffuse (>6 cm). In all three stages, the esophagus maintains its straight profile, whereas in stage IV, in addition to a marked dilation (>6 cm), there is an elongation and angulation of the esophagus, which becomes tortuous and assumes a sigmoid shape (Fig. 17.1). This usually represents the end stage of the disease. The importance of staging lies in the choice of therapy. Stage IV patients treated with a normal laparoscopic Heller myotomy and Dor fundoplication (LHD) showed a less satisfactory outcome than stage I-III patients (76% vs. 88%, respectively) [17]. However, if the lower esophagus is straightened before the LHD by isolating the lower part of the esophagus and verticalizing the organ's axis, the outcome is much better and similar to that of lower stage disease [18] not requiring esophagectomy as the first option.

A modification of the above technique is the timed barium swallow (TBS), in which patients swallow 200 mL of a 45% barium suspension and images are obtained after 1, 2 and 5 min. This enables measurement of the height of the barium

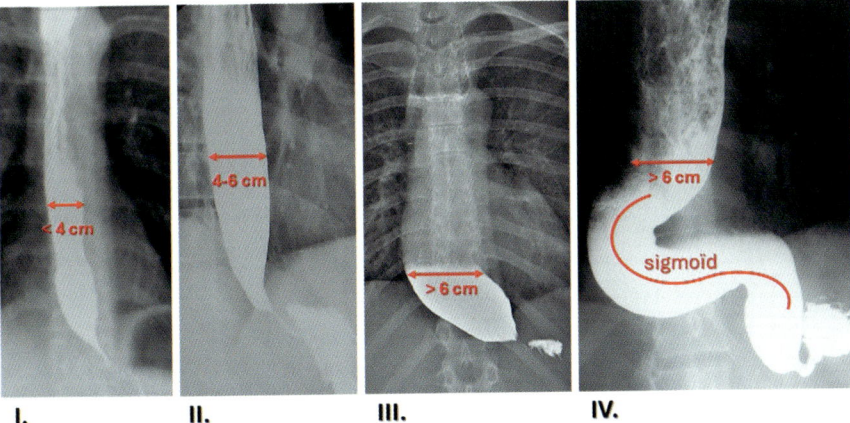

Fig. 17.1 Diagnosis and staging of achalasia with barium swallows. From stage I to stage IV, the esophagus progressively increases in diameter. In stage IV, end-stage disease, it also assumes a sigmoid-like shape

column and of its widest diameter perpendicular to the long axis of the esophagus [19]. The barium empties completely from the esophagus in 1 min in most healthy subjects, and within 5 min in all. Esophageal emptying taking >5 min suggests achalasia [20]. In addition, TBS is most useful and reliable in the objective evaluation of the efficacy of any given treatments of achalasia [21]. The cooperation of an expert radiologist is essential, however, and this may have prevented the wide diffusion of this technique, except in a small number of highly specialized centers.

17.7 Esophageal Manometry

Esophageal manometry has long been the gold standard method for the diagnosis of achalasia. Spechler & Castell [22] defined achalasia by: (1) incomplete or absent relaxation of the LES (with nadir pressure > 8 mmHg) and (2) aperistalsis in the body of the esophagus characterized either by no apparent esophageal contractions or by simultaneous esophageal contractions with amplitudes <40 mmHg, showing a "common cavity phenomenon". A separate rare form of achalasia with some contractions >50–70 mmHg was also reported and called "vigorous achalasia" [23]. This classification lasted unmodified for 30 years.

Then, at the beginning of the new millennium esophageal high-resolution manometry (HRM) was introduced (described in detail in Chap. 4) which, within just a few years revolutionized the field of esophageal motility, making the traditional perfused systems obsolete and possibly inaccurate. This revolution prompted the development of a new classification of esophageal motility disorders, the Chicago Classification (CC), first introduced in 2009 [24]. Updated versions soon followed every few years (CC v2.0 in 2012 [25], and CC v3.0 in 2015 [26]). The aim of this new classification was to standardize the interpretation of HRM, but a

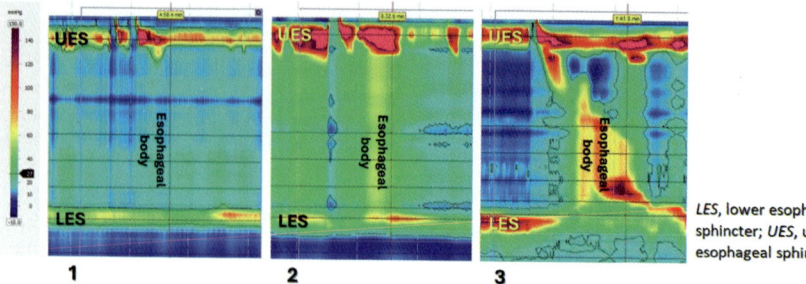

Fig. 17.2 High-resolution manometry (HRM) appearance of achalasia. Within the Chicago Classification, HRM allows the differentiation of the disease in three subtypes. In all of them, impairment of lower esophageal sphincter relaxation on swallowing and absence of peristaltic progression in the esophageal body are pathognomonic. In subtype 1, there is complete absence of pressurization (absent peristalsis) and in subtype 2 substantial pressurization (called pan-pressurization) within the esophagus. In the much less common pattern of vigorous achalasia (subtype 3) there is a spastic contraction within the distal esophageal segment. It is possible that these three subtypes represent different stages in the evolution of the disease rather than different phenotypes

widely accepted consensus was only obtained with CC v3.0, when significant simplification was adopted. Finally, a further, more recent, update that appeared in January 2021 (CC v4.0) [27] recommended the use of both manometric and non-manometric testing to confirm the diagnosis of esophageal motility disorder and the need for a correlation with symptoms before treatment. Since the beginning, achalasia was described with three different body motility patterns: negligible pressurization within the esophagus (absent peristalsis), substantial pressurization (called pan-pressurization) within the esophagus, and a much less common pattern of vigorous achalasia, in which there is a spastic contraction within the distal esophageal segment [24]. Only with CC v2.0, however, were these three different phenotypes "officially" divided into three subtypes [25], based on the recognition that each subtype carried implications for treatment efficacy, subtype 3 being the least responsive to traditional treatments [28]. This classification of achalasia into subtypes was maintained in all the following iterations of the CC (Fig. 17.2).

Moreover, further studies showed that this classification was also possible by carefully reviewing the tracings obtained with traditional manometry [8, 29]. These studies, among others, confirmed the importance of identifying the achalasia subtype in a given patient because there is clear evidence that the subtype is an independent predictor of the success of the various available treatments for achalasia, with subtype 3 having the worst outcome after therapy [1]. In fact, the data from the European Achalasia Trial showed that pneumatic dilation was much less effective in subtype 3 achalasia than in the other subtypes [29]. The same was true in our experience with LHD: when the outcome was stratified by manometric subtypes, patients with subtype 2 had the lowest incidence of failure (4.3%), whereas subtype 1 had a 9.4% failure rate, and subtype 3 a 25% failure rate, $p < 0.001$ [17]. It is possible that in these patients characterized by well-defined, lumen-obliterating spastic contractions in the distal esophagus, reducing the LES pressure (with dilations or surgical myotomy) may not suffice to control the symptoms, especially as the segment affected by the spastic motility extends well above the LES. In this context, peroral endoscopic myotomy (POEM) probably represents a better option [30]. However, since one of our previous studies showed that patients with subtype 3 had a longer LES [8], we modified our classical LHD technique by extending myotomy for 1–2 cm both upwards and downwards, obtaining in these difficult patients an outcome similar to the patients belonging to the other subtypes [31].

It is still not clear whether the three types of achalasia described by the CC are different phenotypes of achalasia or represent different stages in its evolution. Evidence has recently emerged that strongly supports the latter hypothesis, where subtype 3 would be an early stage, subtype 2 an intermediate stage, and subtype 1 the end stage of achalasia [32]. Some cases of transition from one type to another, or from a different motor disorder (distal esophageal spasm, EGJ outflow obstruction) to achalasia have also been described, further supporting the hypothesis labeled as the "Padova theory" (from the group that first suggested it) [33].

References

1. Boeckxstaens GE, Zaninotto G, Richter JE. Achalasia. Lancet. 2014;383(9911):83–93.
2. Hertz AF. Achalasia of the cardia (so-called cardio-spasm). Proc R Soc Med. 1915;8(Clin Sect):22–5.
3. Polonsky L, Guth PH. Familial achalasia. Am J Dig Dis. 1970;15(3):291–5.
4. Savarino E, Bhatia S, Roman S, et al. Achalasia. Nat Rev Dis Primers. 2022;8(1):28.
5. Facco M, Brun P, Baesso I, et al. T cells in the myenteric plexus of achalasia patients show a skewed TCR repertoire and react to HSV-1 antigens. Am J Gastroenterol. 2008;103(7):1598–609.
6. Furuzawa-Carballeda J, Icaza-Chávez ME, Aguilar-León D, et al. Is the Sars-CoV-2 virus a possible trigger agent for the development of achalasia? Neurogastroenterol Motil. 2023;35(3):e14502.
7. Eckardt VF, Aignherr C, Bernhard G. Predictors of outcome in patients with achalasia treated by pneumatic dilation. Gastroenterology. 1992;103(6):1732–8.
8. Salvador R, Costantini M, Zaninotto G, et al. The preoperative manometric pattern predicts the outcome of surgical treatment for esophageal achalasia. J Gastrointest Surg. 2010;14(11):1635–45.
9. Spechler SJ, Souza RF, Rosenberg SJ, et al. Heartburn in patients with achalasia. Gut. 1995;37(3):305–8.
10. Kessing BF, Bredenoord AJ, Smout AJ. Erroneous diagnosis of gastro-esophageal reflux disease in achalasia. Clin Gastroenterol Hepatol. 2011;9(12):1020–4.
11. Müller M, Förschler S, Wehrmann T, et al. Atypical presentations and pitfalls of achalasia. Dis Esophagus. 2023;36(10):doad029.
12. Däbritz J, Domagk D, Monninger M, Foell D. Achalasia mistaken as eating disorders: report of two children and review of the literature. Eur J Gastroenterol Hepatol. 2010;22(7):775–8.
13. El-Takli I, O'Brien P, Paterson WG. Clinical diagnosis of achalasia: how reliable is the barium x-ray? Can J Gastroenterol. 2006;20(5):335–7.
14. Orlando RC, Call DL, Bream CA. Achalasia and absent gastric air bubble. Ann Intern Med. 1978;88(1):60–1.
15. Olsen AM, Holman CB, Andersen HA. The diagnosis of cardiospasm. Dis Chest. 1953;23(5):477–98.

16. Fisichella PM, Raz D, Palazzo F, et al. Clinical, radiological, and manometric profile in 145 patients with untreated achalasia. World J Surg. 2008;32(9):1974–9.
17. Costantini M, Salvador R, Capovilla G, et al. A thousand and one laparoscopic Heller myotomies for esophageal achalasia: a 25-year experience at a single tertiary center. J Gastrointest Surg. 2019;23(1):23–35.
18. Nezi G, Forattini F, Provenzano L, et al. The esophageal pull-down technique improves the outcome of laparoscopic Heller-dor myotomy in end-stage achalasia. J Gastrointest Surg. 2024;28:651–5.
19. de Oliveira JM, Birgisson S, Doinoff C, et al. Timed barium swallow: a simple technique for evaluating esophageal emptying in patients with achalasia. Am J Roentgenol. 1997;169(2):473–9.
20. Neyaz Z, Gupta M, Ghoshal UC. How to perform and interpret timed barium esophagogram. J Neurogastroenterol Motil. 2013;19(2):251–6.
21. Rohof WO, Lei A, Boeckxstaens GE. Esophageal stasis on a timed barium esophagogram predicts recurrent symptoms in patients with long-standing achalasia. Am J Gastroenterol. 2013;108(1):49–55.
22. Spechler SJ, Castell DO. Classification of oesophageal motility abnormalities. Gut. 2001;49(1):145–51.
23. Sanderson DR, Ellis FH Jr, Schlegel JF, Olsen AM. Syndrome of vigorous achalasia: clinical and physiological observations. Dis Chest. 1967;52(4):508–17.
24. Kahrilas PJ, Ghosh SK, Pandolfino JE. Esophageal motility disorders in terms of pressure topography: the Chicago classification. J Clin Gastroenterol. 2008;42(5):627–35.
25. Bredenoord AJ, Fox M, Kahrilas PJ, et al. Chicago classification criteria of esophageal motility disorders defined in high resolution esophageal pressure topography. Neurogastroenterol Motil. 2012;24(Suppl 1):57–65.
26. Kahrilas PJ, Bredenoord AJ, Fox M, et al. The Chicago classification of esophageal motility disorders, v3.0. Neurogastroenterol Motil. 2015;27(2):160–74.
27. Yadlapati R, Kahrilas PJ, Fox MR, et al. Esophageal motility disorders on high-resolution manometry: Chicago classification version 4.0©. Neurogastroenterol Motil. 2021;33(1):e14058.
28. Pandolfino JE, Kwiatek MA, Nealis T, et al. Achalasia: a new clinically relevant classification by high-resolution manometry. Gastroenterology. 2008;135(5):1526–33.
29. Rohof WO, Salvador R, Annese V, et al. Outcomes of treatment for achalasia depend on manometric subtype. Gastroenterology. 2013;144(4):718–25.
30. Modayil RJ, Zhang X, Rothberg B, et al. Peroral endoscopic myotomy: 10-year outcomes from a large, single-center U.S. series with high follow-up completion and comprehensive analysis of long-term efficacy, safety, objective GERD, and endoscopic functional luminal assessment. Gastrointest Endosc. 2021;94(5):930–42.
31. Salvador R, Provenzano L, Capovilla G, et al. Extending myotomy both downward and upward improves the final outcome in manometric pattern III achalasia patients. J Laparoendosc Adv Surg Tech A. 2020;30(2):97–102.
32. Salvador R, Voltarel G, Savarino E, et al. The natural history of achalasia: evidence of a continuum—"the evolutive pattern theory". Dig Liver Dis. 2018;50(4):342–7.
33. Salvador R, Costantini M, Tolone S, et al. Manometric pattern progression in esophageal achalasia in the era of high-resolution manometry. Ann Transl Med. 2021;9(10):906.

Open Access This chapter is licensed under the terms of the Creative Commons Attribution-NonCommercial 4.0 International License (http://creativecommons.org/licenses/by-nc/4.0/), which permits any noncommercial use, sharing, adaptation, distribution and reproduction in any medium or format, as long as you give appropriate credit to the original author(s) and the source, provide a link to the Creative Commons license and indicate if changes were made.

The images or other third party material in this chapter are included in the chapter's Creative Commons license, unless indicated otherwise in a credit line to the material. If material is not included in the chapter's Creative Commons license and your intended use is not permitted by statutory regulation or exceeds the permitted use, you will need to obtain permission directly from the copyright holder.

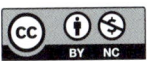

Heller Myotomy and Antireflux Techniques

18

Renato Salvador, Andrea Costantini, Matteo Santangelo, and Salvatore Tolone

18.1 Introduction

At the beginning of the 1990s, minimally invasive techniques were introduced in the clinical treatment of foregut diseases. Because of their advantages in minimizing pain and shortening length of hospital stay, these approaches gained widespread popularity. Laparoscopic Heller myotomy (LHM) for achalasia was first described by Shimi in 1991 [1] and, in 1992, Pellegrini first described the thoracoscopic approach to myotomy [2]. The latter, however, produced abnormal postoperative reflux in as many as 60% of the patients [3] and was thus abandoned. Our group was the first to propose LHM with the addition of a partial anterior fundoplication (Dor), the so-called laparoscopic Heller-Dor operation (LHD) [4]. LHM (and LHD) completely changed the algorithm for the treatment of achalasia, rapidly becoming the procedure of choice, only recently challenged by peroral endoscopic myotomy (POEM) [5].

In this chapter, we describe the technique of LHM, with and without antireflux fundoplication, and discuss the advantages and disadvantages of the different approaches.

R. Salvador (✉) · A. Costantini · M. Santangelo
Department of Surgery, Oncology and Gastroenterology, University of Padua, School of Medicine, Padua, Italy
e-mail: renato.salvador@unipd.it

S. Tolone
UOC General, Mininvasive, Oncological and Bariatric Surgery, University of Campania "Luigi Vanvitelli", Naples, Italy
e-mail: salvatore.tolone@unicampania.it

18.2 Laparoscopic Heller Myotomy (Without Fundoplication)—LHM

The operation is performed under general anesthesia and orotracheal intubation. The patient is placed supine in a reverse Trendelenburg position, with the legs abducted. Moreover, because the poor esophageal emptying due to achalasia causes the esophagus to retain saliva and ingested food, with a high risk of regurgitation and aspiration during anesthesia induction, patients should be kept on a liquid diet for 48 hours before the operation, and the dilated esophagus should be mechanically washed and emptied via a nasoesophageal tube the night before the procedure.

Five trocars are usually used, as in Fig. 18.1.

One assistant on the patient's right side lifts the left liver lobe using an atraumatic retractor, thus exposing the cardia region, whereas one assistant on the patient's left side grasps the gastric fundus, maintaining a caudal traction on the esophagogastric junction. The operation begins with a minimal dissection of the anterior part of the esophagus, thus exposing the anterior esophageal wall. The myotomy is started with the cautery hook 2 cm above the esophagogastric junction to expose the esophageal submucosal layer with the least risk of perforation. The cautery power of the hook is reduced to 15 W to avoid transmitting its coagulating effect to the underlying mucosa. First, the longitudinal muscle fibers are hooked, lifted and coagulated, until the circular fibers are exposed; then the latter are hooked, lifted and divided in the same way. Minor bleeding from the edges of the myotomy can be simply controlled with the aid of mechanical compression using a small sponge. A 6–8 cm long myotomy is performed, extending it on the gastric side to about 2–3 cm, thus exposing the gastric submucosa, which is usually more vascularized than the esophageal one.

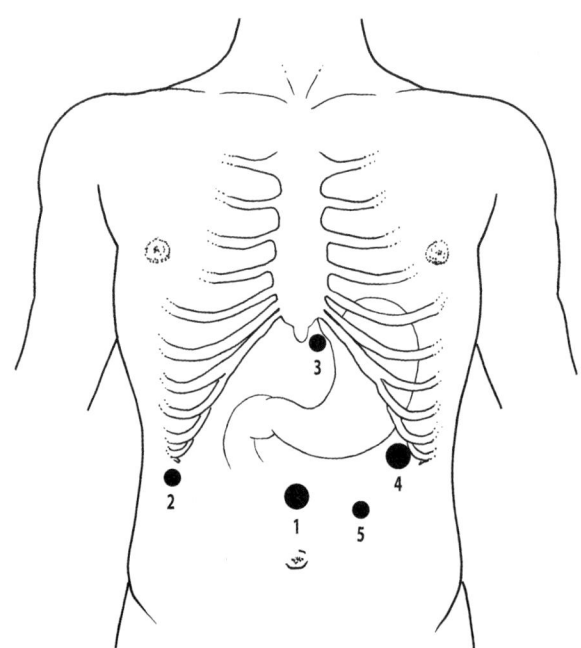

Fig. 18.1 Trocar positioning during Heller-Dor or Heller-Toupet techniques is as follows: (1) supraumbilical (10 mm—for the optic), (2) right hypochondrium (5 mm—for the liver retractor), (3) epigastric (5 mm for the left hand of the first operator), (4) left hypochondrium (10 mm—for the right hand of the first operator, (5) left flank (5 mm—for the third operator). Illustration by Carla Brighenti

Fig. 18.2 A 7–8 cm long myotomy is performed on the esophagus and 2–3 cm on the gastric side. A 30 mm Rigiflex™ balloon, placed inside the esophagus at cardia level, is gently inflated and deflated with 40–60 cc of air using a syringe: this exposes the circular fibers so that they can be stretched and easily cut or torn apart. Illustration by Carla Brighenti

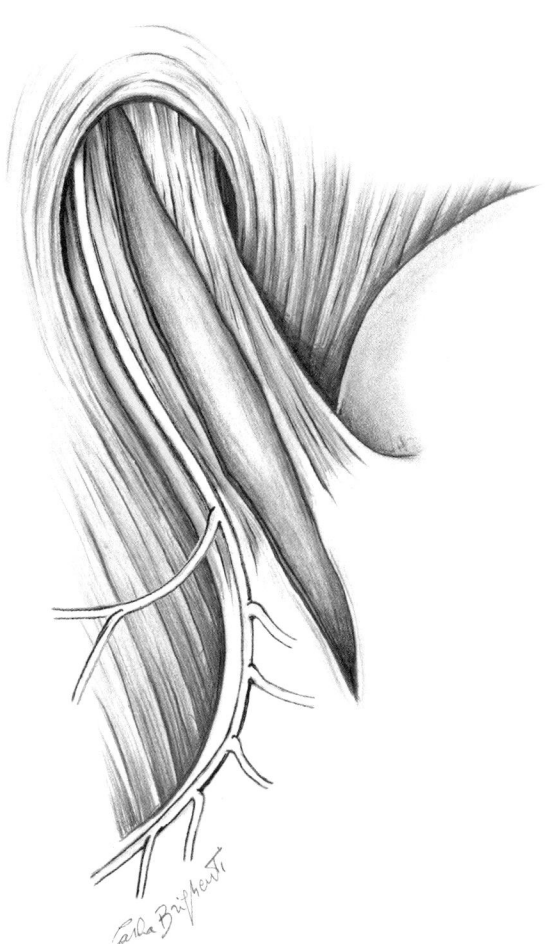

Scissors can be used in the proximal part, whereas hook cautery is used downwards on the gastric side to lift and divide the circular muscle fibers (Fig. 18.2).

Care must be taken during the myotomy to avoid injuring the anterior vagus nerve and to prevent any esophageal perforation of the mucosa. A feature of our personal technique involves the intraoperative use of a 30 mm Rigiflex™ balloon, placed inside the esophagus at cardia level using a guidewire positioned endoscopically before starting the operation. During the myotomy, the balloon is gently inflated and deflated with 30–50 cc of air using a syringe: this exposes the circular fibers so that they can be stretched and easily cut or torn apart.

An esophagogram with a water-soluble contrast (Gastrografin™) is obtained on the first postoperative day to rule out any mucosal perforation. A liquid diet is started, and patients are discharged after another 24–48 hours, once a soft diet has been introduced: this is recommended for 8–10 days, after which a normal diet is allowed. The patients usually return to the outpatients' clinic 2 months later with a barium swallow. As part of our protocol, pH and manometric tests are performed after 6 months, and endoscopy 1one year after the operation [6].

Although some authors only perform the myotomy as described above, a fundoplication is normally added to prevent postoperative gastroesophageal reflux disease (GERD), which may be a severe complication in patients with a poor esophageal clearance due to aperistalsis. Given the lack of peristaltic activity, a partial fundoplication is usually performed, either anteriorly or posteriorly.

In the following paragraphs we briefly describe the most commonly used technique.

18.3 Laparoscopic Heller Myotomy with Dor Fundoplication (LHD)

Laparoscopic Heller-Dor fundoplication (LHD) is the most used technique in tertiary esophageal surgery centers, and involves completing the myotomy with an anterior partial fundoplication according to Dor [6]. With this technique, no posterior dissection is necessary and there is generally no need to mobilize the gastric fundus by dividing the short gastric vessels. An anterior, 180° fundoplication is then made over the esophagus. The fundus is anchored by two rows of stitches on each side of the esophagus, lateral to the exposed mucosa. The proximal left stitch includes the stomach, the edge of the myotomy and the diaphragm (Fig. 18.3). Two

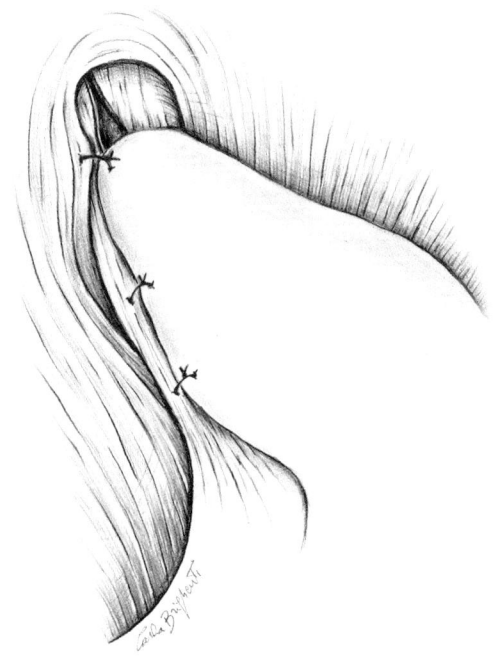

Fig. 18.3 Anterior partial fundoplication following Dor's technique. The fundus is anchored by two rows of stitches on each side of the esophagus, lateral to the exposed mucosa. The proximal left stitch includes the stomach, the edge of the myotomy and the diaphragm. Two or three more stitches are then used to secure the fundus to the left edge of the myotomy. The gastric fundus is then folded over the myotomy, and the greater curvature is anchored to the right pillar and the right edge of the myotomy with three stitches. Illustration by Carla Brighenti

or three more stitches are then used to secure the fundus to the left edge of the myotomy. The gastric fundus is then folded over the myotomy, and the greater curvature is anchored to the right pillar and the right edge of the myotomy with three stitches.

18.4 Laparoscopic Heller Myotomy with Toupet Fundoplication (LHT)

An alternative to the Dor fundoplication is a partial posterior one following Toupet's technique (LHT) [7]. In this case, the operation begins with the opening of the lesser omentum and division of the phrenoesophageal membrane, taking care to preserve the anterior vagus nerve. The greater curvature of the stomach is mobilized, and the esophagus and both vagus nerves are encircled with a Penrose-type drain. With countertraction on the gastroesophageal junction, the dissection is continued liberally into the mediastinum until the gastroesophageal junction remains in the abdomen without tension. After completing the myotomy as described above, a hiatoplasty is usually performed posterior to the esophagus with permanent sutures, to close the esophageal hiatus but avoiding angulation of the esophagus. Then, the gastric fundus is passed through the retroesophageal window, and a 240–270° partial posterior fundoplication is created, anchoring the fundus to the edges of the myotomy to keep them apart. The proximal stitches on both sides usually comprise the corresponding diaphragmatic pillars in addition to the gastric fundus and the edges of the myotomy (Fig. 18.4).

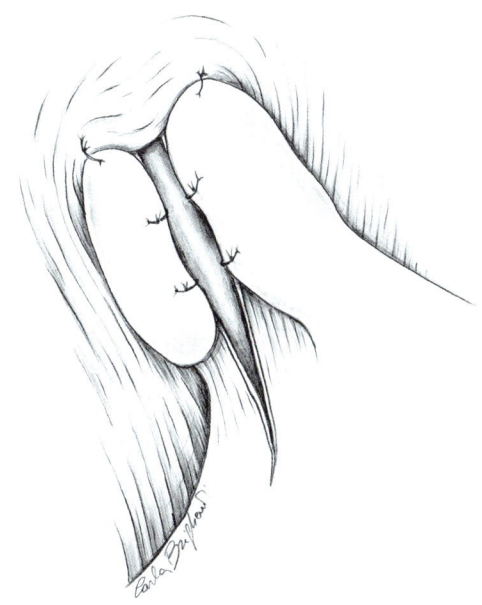

Fig. 18.4 Posterior partial fundoplication following Toupet's technique. After completing the myotomy, the gastric fundus is passed behind the esophagus, completely isolated, through a newly created retroesophageal window, and a 240–270° partial posterior fundoplication is performed, anchoring the fundus to the edges of the myotomy to keep them apart. Illustration by Carla Brighenti

18.5 Laparoscopic Heller Myotomy with Nissen-(Rossetti) Fundoplication (LHN-R)

A total wrap has also been proposed in patients undergoing LHM for achalasia [8]. Also in this case, a wide dissection of the diaphragmatic crura is carried out and the esophagus is widely mobilized on its lower mediastinal and abdominal portion. Taking care to avoid injury to the posterior vagal nerve, a wide retroesophageal space is created behind the lower esophagus, at least 5 cm in length, and the esophagus is gently retracted. Then, after completing the myotomy, a total fundoplication is performed by using the anterior wall of the gastric fundus to perform a 360° Nissen or Nissen-Rossetti fundoplication. The two gastric hemivalves are sutured with two nonabsorbable stitches placed 2 cm apart. The suture does not include the esophageal wall, diaphragmatic pillars or lesser gastric curve. The division of the short gastric vessels is not routinely necessary. More than with the partial fundoplications, this technique needs careful calibration, usually through intraoperative endoscopy and manometry.

18.6 Controversies

18.6.1 To Wrap or Not to Wrap?

The surgical treatment of achalasia carries the risk of triggering the opposite condition, that is, GERD. At present, there are no robust data to demonstrate whether a prophylactic antireflux procedure should be added to the myotomy and, if so, which type of fundoplication is most suitable. Early studies reported conflicting results but were highly flawed for their retrospective nature and the small numbers of patients studied.

A large-scale meta-analysis that reviewed studies reporting on more than 3000 patients gave some definitive insights into this old controversy [9]. In fact, it showed that the incidence of postoperative GERD symptoms was clearly lower if a fundoplication was added to the myotomy (9%) compared to when this was omitted (32%), and the same was especially true when evaluating only the studies which used pH-monitoring to evaluate postoperative reflux (14.5% vs. 41.5%, with or without fundoplication, respectively). Of interest, the rate of GERD after a myotomy without fundoplication were very similar to those now observed after POEM [10].

To date, there are only two randomized controlled trials (RCTs) analyzing outcomes in patients with or without fundoplication after LHM. Falkenback et al. [11] ran a prospective RCT in open Heller myotomy comparing 10 patients with and 10 without associated total fundoplication (floppy Nissen). At >3 years of follow-up, the authors found pathologic GERD by pH testing in 13.1% of the no fundoplication group and in 0.15% of the fundoplication group. No differences in terms of postoperative dysphagia were observed. The RCT by Richards et al. on 43 patients (21 undergoing LHM and 22 LHD) proved the superiority of LHD versus LHM alone regarding postoperative pH-proven GERD (48% vs. 9.5%) [12]. Again, these studies are flawed by the small number of enrolled patients. This may be particularly true for the latter group since, when reporting the late results of their trial [13], the authors were able to contact only 27 of the 41 living patients 12 years after the operation. They showed median dysphagia scores and GERD-health-related quality of life (GERD-HRQL) scores slightly worse for LHM than LHD, without reaching statistical difference, however. Moreover, no pH-studies were performed on this occasion.

More recently, attention was paid to the so-called "limited hiatal dissection", that is, exposure of the anterior wall of the esophagus only. At least three studies [14–16] evaluated the outcome of patients with limited hiatal dissection compared with total dissection, with or without fundoplication. These studies showed that LHM with limited hiatal dissection, as opposed to complete dissection, does not expose the patients to a higher risk of postoperative reflux, irrespective of the addition of a Dor fundoplication.

Finally, it is generally believed today that a laparoscopic short myotomy, usually associated with an inadequate extension onto the gastric wall, is often associated with persistent or recurrent dysphagia [17, 18]. Therefore, most surgeons perform a long myotomy which extends for 2 to 3 cm onto the gastric wall, as originally described by Heller. In this situation, a fundoplication becomes mandatory to prevent postoperative reflux.

In conclusion, the current best practice for the surgical treatment of achalasia is LHM with the addition of a fundoplication, and it is considered in most centers worldwide as the gold standard modality for the approach to achalasia.

18.6.2 Which Fundoplication?

18.6.2.1 Total or Partial?

A total wrap has been proposed in patients undergoing LHM for achalasia. This procedure was particularly favored by an Italian group: Di Martino et al. [19] performed a retrospective comparative study between patients who had anterior partial versus posterior total fundoplication after LHM. After a 2-year follow-up, they reported similar GERD and dysphagia symptom scores. However, Rebecchi et al. ran an RCT analyzing the difference between anterior partial fundoplication to total fundoplication after LHM on 144 patients (72 Dor and 72 Nissen) [20]. At a 5-year follow-up, the incidence of GERD was low and similar in the two groups, but 15% of patients after Nissen fundoplication had dysphagia, as compared with only 2.8% after Dor fundoplication. Because of the lack of peristalsis in achalasia patients, most authors discourage a 360° fundoplication after LHM, since it would increase the outflow resistance, impeding esophageal emptying and causing persistent or recurrent dysphagia. As stated by all the current international guidelines on achalasia [21–23], an LHM with partial wrap (either anterior or posterior) should be the chosen technique for patients with achalasia.

18.6.2.2 Partial Anterior or Posterior?

There is no consensus on what type of partial fundoplication is most effective after LHM. Some surgeons prefer the partial posterior fundoplication (Toupet) because it keeps the edges of the myotomy separated, thus reducing the probability of fibrosis and recurrent dysphagia, and may provide better reflux control. Other experts suggest that the use of a partial anterior fundoplication (Dor) allows limited esophageal dissection thus avoiding disruption of the natural anatomic structures that help control reflux and also allowing a good protection of the exposed mucosa. To date, several RCTs and one meta-analysis have addressed this question. Rawlings et al. [24] published in 2012 a multicenter prospective trial comparing patients undergoing either an anterior or posterior partial wrap after LHM. At 1-year follow-up they found a minimal difference in symptom control between the two groups, whereas 24-hour pH-monitoring showed abnormal reflux more frequently in the Dor group, albeit without reaching statistical significance. Similarly, Kumagai et al. [25] found no significant difference in the Eckardt score or postoperative GERD at 1-year follow-up between patients who had a Dor (n = 20) or a Toupet (n = 22) fundoplication after LHM. Torres et al. compared 38 patients undergoing Dor to 35 undergoing Toupet to complete LHM and showed at 6 months a much lower reflux rate after a Dor (6.9%) than after a Toupet procedure (34%). This difference was confirmed at a longer follow-up (24 months), albeit without reaching statistical significance (10.5% vs. 31.5%, respectively) [26]. Finally, in addition to the already cited meta-analysis by Campos et al. [9], some other meta-analyses recently appeared in literature [27–29], all confirming the substantial equivalence of Dor and Toupet fundoplications as far as reflux control after LHM was concerned.

In conclusion, current evidence fails to demonstrate any significant difference between partial anterior and posterior fundoplication. For the time being, the choice to perform a Dor or a Toupet fundoplication is left to the surgeon's experience and preference. Table 18.1 summarized the advantages and disadvantages of the different types of fundoplications (total and partial, anterior or posterior) usually associated to esophageal myotomy.

Table 18.1 Advantages and disadvantages of different types of fundoplications usually associated with esophageal myotomy

1. Partial fundoplications		
Dor (180°, anterior)		
Pros	Cons	Notes
Isolation of the anterior esophageal wall only. Usually, no need for division of some short gastric vessels. Good protection of the myotomy in case of mucosal lesions, leakage or reoperation.	Dedicated surgical skills.	Recommended (used by most surgeons).
Toupet (270°, posterior)		
Pros	Cons	Notes
Probably better reflux control. Keeps the edges of myotomy well separated. Not indicated in case of mucosal lesions.	Complete isolation of the esophagus, with disruption of all the natural antireflux mechanisms. Possible need for division of some short gastric vessels. No protection of the myotomy.	Recommended (depending on the surgeon's experience).
2. Complete fundoplication		
Nissen (360°, posterior)		
Pros	Cons	Notes
Excellent reflux control.	Postoperative dysphagia. Complete isolation of the esophagus, with disruption of all the natural antireflux mechanisms. Need for division of some short gastric vessels.	Not recommended.

18.7 Peroral Endoscopic Myotomy (POEM) for Achalasia

Achalasia is a rare esophageal motility disorder characterized by impaired relaxation of the lower esophageal sphincter (LES) and absent peristalsis, leading to progressive dysphagia, regurgitation, chest pain, and weight loss. Traditional treatment modalities include pneumatic dilation and Heller myotomy, with the intent of relieving the dysphagia and the outflow obstruction to foods and liquids by lowering the barrier function of the esophagogastric junction. Recently the advent of POEM has revolutionized the management of achalasia by providing a new effective alternative. The mainstay of POEM is the third-space approach; thanks to the ability to create via endoscopy a submucosal tunnel, myotomy can be performed. First introduced in 2010, POEM has since gained widespread acceptance as a primary treatment for achalasia, demonstrating excellent efficacy and safety outcomes [30].

18.7.1 POEM Procedure

POEM is performed under general anesthesia with carbon dioxide insufflation to reduce the risk of complications such as pneumomediastinum or subcutaneous emphysema. The procedure typically lasts 60 to 120 minutes, and most patients can resume oral intake within 24 hours. The procedure consists of four main steps:

1. Mucosal entry—After an initial endoscopic check to assess the esophageal and gastric lumen and verify its axial length, the site of the tunnel entry is decided. Usually, the entry site is located in the posterior wall of the esophagus, so as to avoid accidental pneumoperitoneum. This approach is also useful in the case of re-intervention, in which a previous myotomy is often located anteriorly. Then a saline and methylene blue solution is injected with a water jet injector, in order to create a lifting of the submucosal space. A small incision is then made in the esophageal mucosa using an endoscopic knife.
2. Submucosal tunneling—A cap is usually placed on the tip of the endoscope, which can be useful to lift the submucosal space obtaining a distance between the operative field and the endoscope lens. By alternating water jet infusion and endoscopic knife, a tunnel is created within the submucosal space, extending usually 10 cm above the LES into the proximal stomach. Submucosal vessels are coagulated to avoid bleeding that can hinder correct endoscopic vision.
3. Myotomy—A long myotomy is performed. Depending on the endoscopist's preference, a selective (only circular) or full-thickness myotomy of the muscle layer is performed to relieve the esophageal outflow obstruction. The correct extent and length are debated, although the advantage of offering a longer myotomy than used in the surgical approach in spastic motor disorders is evident.
4. Closure—Finally, the mucosal incision is closed using endoscopic clips or suturing devices to prevent leakage [31]. The patient is allowed to drink and eat few hours after the procedure. Some authors advocate the need for a routine postoperative swallow study in order to assess for leakages.

18.7.2 Efficacy and Safety of POEM

Several studies have demonstrated the effectiveness of POEM in treating achalasia. According to a meta-analysis by Repici et al. [32], POEM achieved clinical success (defined as an Eckardt score ≤ 3) in 92–98% of patients, with sustained symptom relief over long-term follow-up. POEM is effective across all achalasia subtypes (types I, II, and III), including spastic variants that respond poorly to Heller myotomy [33].

While POEM is highly effective, potential adverse effects include GERD, subcutaneous emphysema, and mucosal injuries. GERD is the most common post-procedure complication, affecting up to 40% of patients and necessitating long-term proton-pump inhibitor therapy [34]. This complication is intuitive; achieving a good myotomy, as POEM allows, means that the esophagogastric junction barrier no longer opposes the outflow of what a patient has swallowed, but it should not anymore be effective against reflux. Thus, how best to select patients for POEM or Heller myotomy is still debated.

18.7.3 Comparison with Heller Myotomy and Pneumatic Dilation

Compared to LHM, POEM offers similar symptom relief and similar hospital stays and recovery [35]. Unlike LHM, POEM allows for individualized myotomy lengths, making it preferable for type III achalasia. Compared to pneumatic dilation, POEM has a significantly lower risk of symptom recurrence, making it the superior long-term treatment choice [36].

18.8 Conclusions

Current evidence and all the recent guidelines on the treatment of achalasia confirm that laparoscopic myotomy is a safe and effective long-term treatment, and that the addition of a partial fundoplication leads to a lower rate of postoperative reflux without compromising esophageal emptying. It should therefore be regarded at the surgical treatment of choice for this condition.

POEM has emerged as a highly effective minimally invasive treatment for achalasia, with excellent outcomes and a favorable safety profile. Despite the risk of GERD, its advantages over traditional treatments make it an effective option for many patients. Ongoing advancements in endoscopic techniques will continue to refine POEM, ensuring improved patient outcomes in the future.

Acknowledgments The authors would like to thank Ms. Carla Brighenti, Department of Surgical, Oncological and Gastrointestinal Sciences University of Padua, for the preparation of the chapter figures.

References

1. Shimi S, Nathanson LK, Cuschieri A. Laparoscopic cardiomyotomy for achalasia. J R Coll Surg Edinb. 1991;36(3):152–4.
2. Pellegrini C, Wetter LA, Patti M, et al. Thoracoscopic esophagomyotomy. Initial experience with a new approach for the treatment of achalasia. Ann Surg. 1992;216(3):291–6.
3. Patti MG, Pellegrini CA, Horgan S, et al. Minimally invasive surgery for achalasia: an 8-year experience with 168 patients. Ann Surg. 1999;230(4):587–93.
4. Ancona E, Peracchia A, Zaninotto G, et al. Heller laparoscopic cardiomyotomy with antireflux anterior fundoplication (Dor) in the treatment of esophageal achalasia. Surg Endosc. 1993;7(5):459–61.
5. Inoue H, Minami H, Kobayashi Y, et al. Peroral endoscopic myotomy (POEM) for esophageal achalasia. Endoscopy. 2010;42(4):265–71.

6. Costantini M, Salvador R, Capovilla G, et al. A thousand and one laparoscopic Heller myotomies for esophageal achalasia: a 25-year experience at a single tertiary center. J Gastrointest Surg. 2019;23(1):23–35.
7. Toupet A. Technique d'oesophago-gastroplastie avec phrénicogastropexie appliquée dan la cure radicale des hernias hiatales et comme complément de l'operation d'Heller dans les cardiospasmes. Mem Acad Chir (Paris). 1963;89:394–9.
8. Patti MG, Robinson T, Galvani C, et al. Total fundoplication is superior to partial fundoplication even when esophageal peristalsis is weak. J Am Coll Surg. 2004;198:863–70.
9. Campos GM, Vittinghoff E, Rabl C, et al. Endoscopic and surgical treatments for achalasia: a systematic review and meta-analysis. Ann Surg. 2009;249:45–57.
10. Repici A, Fuccio L, Maselli R, et al. GERD after per-oral endoscopic myotomy as compared with Heller's myotomy with fundoplication: a systematic review with meta-analysis. Gastrointest Endosc. 2018;87(4):934–943.e18.
11. Falkenback D, Johansson J, Öberg S, et al. Heller's esophagomyotomy with or without a 360° floppy Nissen fundoplication for achalasia. Long-term results from a prospective randomized study. Dis Esophagus. 2003;16:284–90.
12. Richards WO, Torquati A, Holzman MD, et al. Heller myotomy versus Heller myotomy with Dor fundoplication for achalasia: a prospective randomized double-blind clinical trial. Ann Surg. 2004;240(3):405–12.
13. Kummerow Broman K, Phillips SE, Faqih A, et al. Heller myotomy versus Heller myotomy with dor fundoplication for achalasia: long-term symptomatic follow-up of a prospective randomized controlled trial. Surg Endosc. 2018;32(4):1668–74.
14. Robert M, Poncet G, Mion F, Boulez J. Results of laparoscopic Heller myotomy without anti-reflux procedure in achalasia. Monocentric prospective study of 106 cases. Surg Endosc. 2008;22(4):866–74.
15. Simić AP, Radovanović NS, Skrobić OM, et al. Significance of limited hiatal dissection in surgery for achalasia. J Gastrointest Surg. 2010;14:587–93.
16. DeHaan RK, Frelich MJ, Gould JC. Limited hiatal dissection without fundoplication results in comparable symptomatic outcomes to laparoscopic Heller myotomy with anterior fundoplication. J Laparoendosc Adv Surg Tech A. 2016;26(7):506–10.
17. Wright AS, Williams CW, Pellegrini CA, Oelschlager BK. Long term outcomes confirm the superior efficacy of extended Heller myotomy with Toupet fundoplication for achalasia. Surg Endosc. 2007;21(5):713–8.
18. Oelschlager BK, Chang L, Pellegrini CA. Improved outcome after extended gastric myotomy for achalasia. Arch Surg. 2003;138(5):490–5.
19. Di Martino N, Brillantino A, Monaco L, et al. Laparoscopic calibrated total vs partial fundoplication following heller myotomy for oesophageal achalasia. World J Gastroenterol. 2011;17:3431–40.
20. Rebecchi F, Giaccone C, Farinella E, et al. Randomized controlled trial of laparoscopic heller myotomy plus Dor fundoplication versus Nissen fundoplication for achalasia long-term results. Ann Surg. 2008;248:1023–9.
21. Zaninotto G, Bennett C, Boeckxstaens G, et al. The 2018 ISDE achalasia guidelines. Dis Esophagus. 2018 Sep 1;31(9)
22. Oude Nijhuis RAB, Zaninotto G, Roman S, et al. European guidelines on achalasia: united European gastroenterology and European Society of Neurogastroenterology and Motility recommendations. United European Gastroenterol J. 2020;8(1):13–33.
23. Vaezi MF, Pandolfino JE, Yadlapati RH, et al. ACG clinical guidelines: diagnosis and management of achalasia. Am J Gastroenterol. 2020;115(9):1393–411.
24. Rawlings A, Soper N, Oelschlager B. Laparoscopic Dor versus Toupet fundoplication following Heller myotomy for achalasia: results of a multicenter, prospective randomized-controlled trial. Surg Endosc. 2012;26(1):18–26.
25. Kumagai K, Kjellin A, Tsai JA, et al. Toupet versus Dor as a procedure to prevent reflux after cardiomyotomy for achalasia: results of a randomised clinical trial. Int J Surg. 2014;12:673–80.

26. Torres-Villalobos G, Coss-Adame E, Furuzawa-Carballeda J, et al. Dor vs Toupet fundoplication after laparoscopic Heller myotomy: long-term randomized controlled trial evaluated by high-resolution manometry. J Gastrointest Surg. 2018;22(1):13–22.
27. Kurian AA, Bhayani N, Sharata A, et al. Partial anterior vs partial posterior fundoplication following transabdominal esophagocardiomyotomy for achalasia of the esophagus: meta-regression of objective postoperative gastroesophageal reflux and dysphagia. JAMA Surg. 2013;148(1):85–90.
28. Aiolfi A, Tornese S, Bonitta G, et al. Dor versus Toupet fundoplication after laparoscopic Heller myotomy: systematic review and bayesian meta-analysis of randomized controlled trials. Asian J Surg. 2020;43(1):20–8.
29. Santoro G, Sheriff N, Noronha J, et al. Heller myotomy versus Heller myotomy with fundoplication in patients with achalasia: a systematic review and meta-analysis. Ann R Coll Surg Engl. 2022;104(3):158–64.
30. Inoue H, Minami H, Kobayashi Y, et al. Peroral endoscopic myotomy for esophageal achalasia: a prospective multicenter study. Ann Surg. 2010;252(1):90–6.
31. Li H, Peng W, Huang S, et al. Efficacy and safety of peroral endoscopic myotomy for achalasia: a systematic review and meta-analysis. J Gastroenterol Hepatol. 2019;34(6):985–95.
32. Repici A, Fuccio L, Maselli R, et al. Peroral endoscopic myotomy for achalasia: long-term results of a European multicenter study. Endoscopy. 2018;50(6):575–82.
33. Bechara R, Onimaru M, Ikeda H, Inoue H. Peroral endoscopic myotomy: achievements and perspectives. Clin Endosc. 2016;49(6):521–9.
34. Shiwaku H, Inoue H, Yamashita K, et al. Peroral endoscopic myotomy for type III achalasia: outcomes and technical modifications. Surg Endosc. 2021;35(3):1098–107.
35. Werner YB, Costamagna G, Swanström LL, et al. Endoscopic or surgical myotomy in patients with idiopathic achalasia. N Engl J Med. 2019;381(23):2219–29.
36. Zhang X, Zhang W, Li Q, et al. Peroral endoscopic myotomy versus laparoscopic Heller myotomy for achalasia: a systematic review and meta-analysis. J Dig Dis. 2020;21(7):374–82.

Open Access This chapter is licensed under the terms of the Creative Commons Attribution-NonCommercial 4.0 International License (http://creativecommons.org/licenses/by-nc/4.0/), which permits any noncommercial use, sharing, adaptation, distribution and reproduction in any medium or format, as long as you give appropriate credit to the original author(s) and the source, provide a link to the Creative Commons license and indicate if changes were made.

The images or other third party material in this chapter are included in the chapter's Creative Commons license, unless indicated otherwise in a credit line to the material. If material is not included in the chapter's Creative Commons license and your intended use is not permitted by statutory regulation or exceeds the permitted use, you will need to obtain permission directly from the copyright holder.

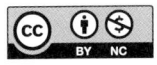

Pharyngoesophageal Diverticula

Luigi Bonavina

19.1 Introduction

Zenker diverticulum (ZD) is an acquired mucosal pouch protruding from the posterior aspect of the pharyngoesophageal junction (Killian's triangle). Pathogenetic factors include altered upper esophageal sphincter coordination, increased intrabolus pressure, and reduced hypopharyngeal wall compliance [1, 2]. ZD is considered a rare disease, with a prevalence of 0.11% or 2/100,000 persons/year, but the incidence is likely to increase in the future due to progressive population aging [3]. It is currently estimated that the annual case-load in referral centers is 8.7 patients per year [4]. Common presenting symptoms are dysphagia and regurgitation, and the most frequent complication is recurrent aspiration pneumonia [5].

Historically, surgical treatment consisted of surgical resection of the pouch. During the last five decades, the crucial role of the cricopharyngeal muscle has been recognized and cricopharyngeal myotomy, performed either surgically or endoscopically, has become the main target of treatment. This attitude reflects a better understanding of the pathophysiology of the disease and the need to minimize recurrence rates and improve quality of life in these patients [6–8]. Nowadays, the development of minimally invasive technologies has driven profound changes in management culminating in the introduction of Zenker peroral endoscopic myotomy (Z-POEM).

L. Bonavina (✉)
Department of Biomedical Sciences for Health, University of Milan, Milan, Italy

Division of General and Foregut Surgery, IRCCS Policlinico San Donato, San Donato Milanese, Italy
e-mail: luigi.bonavina@unimi.it

19.2 Shift from Open Access to Transoral Surgery

Initially, ZD was treated by open surgery or rigid endoscopy with the aim, respectively, of resecting the pouch or dividing the septum between the esophagus and the diverticulum. The importance of adding a cricopharyngeal myotomy to surgical resection of the pouch was increasingly recognized as a critical component of the procedure to minimize leaks and symptomatic recurrences. This has encouraged the development of minimally invasive transoral techniques to divide the common septum using electrocautery or CO_2 laser [9]. In 1993, at the beginning of the laparoscopic era, endostaplers were introduced to standardize and make safer the procedure of septal division [10–12]. The technique showed excellent clinical outcomes especially in patients with medium- or large-sized (3–6 cm) diverticula. Manometric and scintigraphic studies confirmed restoration of pharyngoesophageal physiology with decrease of hypopharyngeal intrabolus pressure and improved pharyngeal clearance [13]. However, placement of the rigid Weerda diverticuloscope and actioning of the endostapler might be difficult in patients with neck stiffness or limited mouth opening [14, 15]. In addition, the procedure is not suitable for individuals with small diverticula (<3 cm) because of the inability to engage enough cricopharyngeal muscle tissue for stapling across the entire septum length [16, 17]. A multicenter study on 585 patients operated on by otolaryngologists showed a conversion rate of 7.7%, an overall complication rate of 9.6%, and a recurrence rate of 12.8% [18]. Over the years, a modified endostapling technique using a traction suture on the apex of the septum has been proposed to add an average 1 cm of septum length into the stapler jaws, thus enabling extended septal division [19, 20]. In addition, a variety of cutting and coagulation devices, including Harmonic scalpel and LigaSure, have been introduced to provide complete distal septum division over the uncut suture line. Soft overtubes have also been proposed to obviate the difficulties in positioning the rigid diverticuloscope [21].

19.3 Shift from Standard Flexible Endoscopy to Third-Space Endoscopy

Although transoral stapling was the preferred initial approach for ZD, lack of expertise with the rigid diverticuloscope, anatomic limitations of septum exposure such as reduced neck extension or inadequate mouth opening, and the requirement for narcosis encouraged the development of flexible endoscopic septotomy (FES) in 1995 [22]. Since then, this procedure has commonly been performed under deep sedation and in the outpatient setting, thus allowing the treatment of elderly patients with small (<3 cm) pouches who may be unfit for general anesthesia. Different devices such as needle-knife, hook-knife, harmonic scalpel, laser, etc. have been used to perform FES with satisfactory outcomes. Use of CO_2 insufflation and routine mucosal closure have been consistently recommended to minimize the risk of perforation. Regardless of the device used, FES has proven feasible and effective during short-term follow-up, with an average recurrence rate of 29% [23–25]. The FES procedure is repeatable, and multiple treatments can be done to complete septum division. Despite early enthusiasm with the flexible endoscopic techniques, a systematic review and network meta-analysis including 903 patients and comparing endoscopic laser-assisted diverticulotomy, endoscopic stapler-assisted diverticulotomy, and transcervical diverticulectomy, concluded that the open surgical approach has a decreased likelihood of persistent or recurrent symptoms compared with the endoscopic techniques [26].

Experience with the use of POEM for esophageal achalasia has helped to translate the principles of third-space endoscopy to the pharyngoesophageal area, thereby pushing the boundaries of both transoral stapling and FES [27]. The technique of Z-POEM allows cricopharyngeal myotomy through submucosal tunneling. The majority of reports now differentiate between two different tunneling techniques based on the site of mucosal incision. In the conventional technique, the hypopharyngeal mucosa is opened 1.5–2 cm proximal to the septum and the submucosal tunneling is created to reach and divide the cricopharyngeal muscle. The mucosal entry site is then closed with endoclips. Performing the incision proximal to the septum makes the procedure safer given its distance from the mediastinum, but care must be taken to avoid tearing the hypopharyngeal mucosa. Other limitations of Z-POEM are that the proximal esophageal muscle is not divided and that the defunctionalized remnant pouch may be responsible for residual symptoms. A recent meta-analysis of 11 studies [28] with 357 patients showed a pooled technical success of 96.3% (95% CI: 93.6–97.9), a pooled incidence of adverse events of 12.4% (95% CI: 9.1–16.7), and a clinical success rate of 93% (95% CI: 89.4–95.4). The pooled clinical recurrence rate was 11.2% (95% CI: 7.6–16.2).

An alternative third-space approach, called Zenker peroral endoscopic septotomy (Z-POES), was developed to overcome the technical challenges of the Z-POEM technique and to improve outcomes. The modified tunneling technique consists of opening the mucosa on top of the long axis of the septum to gain direct access to the muscle. Then, the submucosal tunnel ahead and behind the cricopharyngeal muscle is created and the proximal esophageal muscle fibers are divided [29]. At the end of the myotomy, a remodeling septoplasty can be performed to prevent a large residual pouch [30].

A recent pilot study on 20 patients advocated the use of Z-POES for ZD >20 mm in size [31]. The average procedural time was 13.8 min, and the technique was successful in 100% of patients. No symptomatic adverse events occurred, and the 1-year clinical success rate was 95%. In a recent systematic review [32], which included nine studies and a total of 196 patients undergoing Z-POEM or Z-POES, the pooled rate of clinical success and adverse events was 93.4% and 4.9%, respectively, with no significant differences in terms of efficacy and safety between the two tunneling techniques.

At our esophageal center, a total of 271 patients have been treated for ZD over the past two decades. Of these individuals, 198 (73%) underwent transoral stapling through rigid endoscopy, 53 (19.6%) patients underwent a flexible endoscopic procedure (36 FES and 17 Z-POES), and only 20 (7.4%) patients underwent open surgery. The technical and clinical success rate of Z-POES were 100% and 94.2%, respectively. One patient developed a subclinical leak which was treated conservatively with antibiotics and naso-enteral nutrition [33].

19.4 Management of Recurrent Zenker Diverticulum

Symptoms of ZD may recur regardless of the primary treatment modality, with recurrence rates ranging from 4.2% after open surgery to 18.4% after endoscopic therapy [25]. The management of recurrent ZD varies widely, but reported data are limited. The choice of the revisional technique depends on patient age, comorbidities, pouch size, and surgeon preference and expertise. In a retrospective multicenter study with 56 patients, the index procedure was open surgery in 30% and endoscopic in 70%. Revisional procedures were performed open in 37.5% of cases and endoscopically in 62.5% after an average time of 4.6 years after the primary treatment. Both procedures were reported to be safe and effective [34].

19.5 Comment

A complete cricopharyngeal myotomy represents the cornerstone of therapy for ZD. The development of transoral techniques has allowed a minimally invasive and precision approach. Indeed, patient's anatomical characteristics, small pouches, and lack of physician's expertise with rigid endoscopy represent significant limitations of the classical transoral stapling technique. Conversely, submucosal endoscopic procedures appear safe and effective, providing excellent exposure of the cricopharyngeal septum and muscle, and allowing for a precise single-stage myotomy with possible pouch remodeling. This may translate into reduction of anatomical and symptomatic recurrences and lower reintervention rates.

Management of ZD requires an interdisciplinary and cooperative approach of multiple specialists (foregut surgeons, gastroenterologists, and otolaryngologists) to deliver the best care to the patient. Nowadays, indications for an open surgical approach have become rare. In our opinion, large ZD (>3 cm) can be safely treated with endostapling, and smaller or recurrent ZD should be treated with Z-POES.

In conclusion, a tailored approach is feasible and safe in tertiary-care hospitals. POEM techniques have indeed opened a new era in the management of ZD and may soon become the first-line approach. Appropriate training in advanced operative endoscopy remains a critical issue. High-quality studies with standardized patient-reported outcomes and long-term follow-up are necessary to validate these very promising clinical findings.

Acknowledgments This chapter is in part based on the following article: Scardino A, Siboni S, Milito P, Bonavina L. Expanding the therapeutic options for Zenker's diverticulum: from open diverticulectomy to transoral septoplasty. Mini-invasive Surg. 2022;6:57. https://doi.org/10.20517/2574-1225.2022.55. This is an open access article distributed under the terms and conditions of the Creative Commons Attribution (CC BY) license (https://creativecommons.org/licenses/by/4.0/).

References

1. Bonavina L, Khan NA, DeMeester TR, Pharyngoesophageal dysfunctions. The role of cricopharyngeal myotomy. Arch Surg. 1985;120(5):541–9.
2. Cook IJ, Gabb M, Panagopoulos V, et al. Pharyngeal (Zenker's) diverticulum is a disorder of upper esophageal sphincter opening. Gastroenterology. 1992;103:1229–35.
3. Law R, Katzka DA, Baron TH. Zenker's diverticulum. Clin Gastroenterol Hepatol. 2014;12:1773–82.
4. Nitschke P, Kemper M, Konig P, et al. Interdisciplinary comparison of endoscopic laser-assisted diverticulotomy vs. transcervical myotomy as a treatment for Zenker's diverticulum. J Gastrointest Surg. 2020;24(9):1955–61.
5. Siboni S, Asti E, Sozzi M, et al. Respiratory symptoms and complications of Zenker diverticulum: effect of trans-oral septum stapling. J Gastrointest Surg. 2017;21(9):1391–5.
6. Bonavina L. Surgical management of esophageal diverticula. In: Yeo CJ, editor. Shackelford's surgery of the alimentary tract, vol. 1. Saunders Elsevier; 2007. p. 427–40.
7. Aiolfi A, Scolari F, Saino G, Bonavina L. Current status of minimally invasive endoscopic management for Zenker diverticulum. World J Gastrointest Endosc. 2015;7(2):87–93.
8. Bonavina L, Bona D, Abraham M, et al. Long-term results of endosurgical and open surgical approach for Zenker diverticulum. World J Gastroenterol. 2007;13(18):2586–9.
9. Van Overbeek JJM. Pathogenesis and methods of treatment of Zenker's diverticulum. Ann Otol Rhinol Laryngol. 2003;112(7):583–93.
10. Collard JM, Otte JB, Kestens PJ. Endoscopic stapling technique of esophagodiverticulostomy for Zenker's diverticulum. Ann Thorac Surg. 1993;56(3):573–6.
11. Martin-Hirsch DP, Newbegin CJ. Autosuture GIA gun: a new application in the treatment of hypopharyngeal diverticula. J Laryngol Otol. 1993;107:723–5.
12. Narne S, Bonavina L, Guido E, Peracchia A. Treatment of Zenker's diverticulum by endoscopic stapling. Endosurgery. 1993;1:118–20.
13. Peracchia A, Bonavina L, Narne S, et al. Minimally invasive surgery for Zenker diverticulum: analysis of results in 95 consecutive patients. Arch Surg. 1998;133(7):695–700.
14. Bloom JD, Bleier BS, Mirza N, et al. Factors predicting endoscopic exposure of Zenker's diverticulum. Ann Otol Rhinol Laryngol. 2010;119(11):736–41.
15. Milito P, Siboni S, Asti E, Bonavina L. Anthropometric variables predict feasibility and long-term outcomes of trans-oral septum stapling for Zenker diverticulum. J Gastrointest Surg. 2023;27(3):590–3.
16. Narne S, Cutrone C, Bonavina L, et al. Endoscopic diverticulotomy for the treatment of Zenker's diverticulum: results in 102 patients with staple-assisted endoscopy. Ann Otol Rhinol Laryngol. 1999;108(8):810–5.
17. Tsikoudas A, Eason D, Kara N, et al. Correlation of radiologic findings and clinical outcome in pharyngeal pouch stapling. Ann Otol Rhinol Laryngol. 2006;115(10):721–6.
18. Leong SC, Wilkie MD, Webb CJ. Endoscopic stapling of Zenker's diverticulum: establishing national baselines for auditing clinical outcomes in the United Kingdom. Eur Arch Otorrinolaringol. 2012;269:1877–84.

19. Nicholas BD, Devitt S, Rosen D, et al. Endostitch-assisted endoscopic Zenker's diverticulostomy: a tried approach for difficult cases. Dis Esophagus. 2010;23(4):296–9.
20. Bonavina L, Rottoli M, Bona D, et al. Transoral stapling for Zenker diverticulum: effect of the traction suture-assisted technique on long-term outcomes. Surg Endosc. 2012;26(10):2856–61.
21. Bonavina L, Bona D, Aiolfi A, Sironi A. Transoral septum stapling of Zenker diverticulum is feasible and safe through a soft overtube. Surg Innov. 2015;22(2):207–9.
22. Ishioka S, Sakai P, Maluf Filho F, Melo JM. Endoscopic incision of Zenker's diverticula. Endoscopy. 1995;27:433–7.
23. Bizzotto A, Iacopini F, Landi R, Costamagna G. Zenker's diverticulum: exploring treatment options. Acta Otorhinolaryngol Ital. 2013;33(4):219–29.
24. Ishaq S, Hassan C, Antonello A, et al. Flexible endoscopic treatment for Zenker's diverticulum: a systematic review and meta-analysis. Gastrointest Endosc. 2016;83(6):1076–1089.e5.
25. Verdonck J, Morton RP. Systematic review on treatment of Zenker's diverticulum. Eur Arch Otorrinolaringol. 2015;272(11):3095–107.
26. Bhatt NK, Mendoza J, Kallogjeri D, et al. Comparison of surgical treatments for Zenker diverticulum. A systematic review and network meta-analysis. JAMA Otolaryngol Head Neck Surg. 2021;147(2):190–6.
27. Li QL, Chen WF, Zhang XC, et al. Submucosal tunneling endoscopic septum division: a novel technique for treating Zenker's diverticulum. Gastroenterology. 2016;151(6):1071–4.
28. Zhang H, Huang S, Xia H, et al. The role of peroral endoscopic myotomy for Zenker's diverticulum: a systematic review and meta-analysis. Surg Endosc. 2022;36(5):2749–59.
29. Mavrogenis G, Tsevgas I, Zachariadis D, Bazerbachi F. Mucosotomy at the top of the septum facilitates tunneling and clipping during peroral endoscopic myotomy for Zenker's diverticulum (Z-POEM). Ann Gastroenterol. 2020;33(1):101.
30. Zhang LY, Nieto J, Ngamruengphong S, et al. Zenker's diverticulum: advancing beyond the tunnel. VideoGIE. 2021;6:562–7.
31. Repici A, Spadaccini M, Belletrutti PJ, et al. Peroral endoscopic septotomy for short-septum Zenker's diverticulum. Endoscopy. 2020;52(7):563–8.
32. Spadaccini M, Maselli R, Chandrasekar VT, et al. Submucosal tunnelling techniques for Zenker's diverticulum: a systematic review of early outcomes with pooled analysis. Eur J Gastroenterol Hepatol. 2021;33(1S):e78–83.
33. Scardino A, Siboni S, Milito P, Bonavina L. Expanding the therapeutic options for Zenker's diverticulum: from open diverticulectomy to transoral septoplasty. Mini-invasive Surg. 2022;6:57.
34. Berger MH, Weiland D, Tierney S, et al. Surgical management of recurrent Zenker's diverticulum: a multi-institutional cohort study. Am J Otolaryngol. 2021;42(1):102755.

Open Access This chapter is licensed under the terms of the Creative Commons Attribution-NonCommercial 4.0 International License (http://creativecommons.org/licenses/by-nc/4.0/), which permits any noncommercial use, sharing, adaptation, distribution and reproduction in any medium or format, as long as you give appropriate credit to the original author(s) and the source, provide a link to the Creative Commons license and indicate if changes were made.

The images or other third party material in this chapter are included in the chapter's Creative Commons license, unless indicated otherwise in a credit line to the material. If material is not included in the chapter's Creative Commons license and your intended use is not permitted by statutory regulation or exceeds the permitted use, you will need to obtain permission directly from the copyright holder.

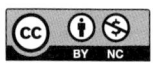

Epiphrenic Diverticula

20

Lavinia Alessandra Barbieri, Silvia Battaglia,
Agnese Carresi, Francesco Puccetti, Ugo Elmore,
and Riccardo Rosati

20.1 Introduction

Esophageal diverticula are a relatively rare condition, potentially developing along the entire length of the esophagus and varying in incidence and etiology for each location.

Epiphrenic diverticula (ED) are located in the lower part of the esophagus, within 10 cm above the cardias and they account for 20% of all esophageal diverticula, and are the second most common after pharyngoesophageal ones.

The real incidence is unknown, given that some of them are discovered incidentally; only 52 cases were reported up to 1952. Radiological studies have shown that ED have a prevalence of 0.015% in the United States and up to 0.77% in Japan and 2.0% in Europe [1].

20.2 Pathophysiology

Also called false or pseudo-diverticula, ED enclose only the mucosal and submucosal lining, herniating through a weakness in the muscularis layer of the esophagus. This anatomical weakness in the muscularis layer is located where the nerves and blood vessels enter to supply the distal esophagus, or at the antimesenteric border of the embryonic foregut esophageal wall [1, 2].

The presence of a motility disorder has been widely reported to affect from 35% to 90% of patients with ED [3]; the most frequently diagnosed disturbance has always been achalasia, mainly detected through the use of conventional manometry to assess esophageal motility. However, other esophageal motility diagnoses, defined by varying

---

L. A. Barbieri · S. Battaglia · A. Carresi · F. Puccetti · U. Elmore · R. Rosati (✉)
IRCCS San Raffaele Scientific Institute and San Raffaele Vita-Salute University, Milan, Italy
e-mail: barbieri.lavinia@hsr.it; battaglia.silvia@hsr.it; carresi.agnese@hsr.it; puccetti.francesco@hsr.it; elmore.ugo@hsr.it; rosati.riccardo@hsr.it

© The Author(s) 2026
V. Landolfi, S. Tolone (eds.), *Functional Diseases of the Esophagus*, Updates in Surgery, https://doi.org/10.1007/978-3-031-90570-4_20

conventional manometry-based criteria and including distal esophageal spasm and nutcracker esophagus have been reported in varying frequencies in patients with esophageal diverticula. Some series, on the other hand, have reported lower rates of a defined esophageal dysmotility; a comprehensive study by the Chicago group observed, by means of high-resolution manometry (HRM) and esophageal pressure topography, abnormal pressurization in the compartmentalization phase often with hypercontractility in patients with mid-thoracic and epiphrenic esophageal diverticula, even in patients with no esophageal motility disturbances [4]. Failure to include treatment of the motility disorder into the management of ED sets the stage for the onset of postoperative complications such as leaks at the suture line or recurrent diverticulum.

Another issue in the diagnostic work-up is the lower technical success of performing HRM in patients suffering from diverticula: in a recent study, HRM was completely successful in 70% of ED patients as compared with 91% of the control group. The reason is mainly the inability to traverse the esophagogastric junction due to the size of the diverticulum [5]. However, this problem might be solved by placing the manometry catheter through endoscopy.

A very special category of ED occurs as a result of iatrogenic damage due to an excessively tight wrap or myotomy for achalasia or, even more frequently, as a complication of peroral endoscopic myotomy (POEM), also known as a "blown-out" myotomy. In these cases, the treatment ranges from pneumatic dilation to a redo fundoplication or redo myotomy depending on the iatrogenic cause [6].

20.3 Clinical Presentation

A large number of diverticula are discovered incidentally and the symptoms can be mild or totally absent. The clinical presentation of ED can be divided into two categories: symptoms related to the underlying motility disorder, such as dysphagia and regurgitation of undigested food or saliva and chest pain, and respiratory complaints due to aspiration such as recurrent pneumonia and dyspnea or pulmonary fibrosis. No correlation between the size of the diverticulum and the severity of these symptoms has been demonstrated [7]. In addition, when the diverticulum becomes large enough, it may also cause dysphagia by extrinsic compression of the distal esophagus. Rarely, the presentation is acute for a complication such as bolus impaction, bleeding or spontaneous rupture [8, 9].

The evolution into carcinoma is extremely rare, with a reported incidence of 0.6% [10]; symptoms of hematemesis or melena are suspicious.

20.4 Preoperative Work-Up

A barium esophagogram is typically the first diagnostic test performed (Fig. 20.1). It is mandatory for careful planning of surgery: it is necessary to look for any additional diverticula to the larger one, and assess the esophageal side of the pouch that will drive the stapler application, the distance from cardias, and the dimension of the diverticular pouch and neck.

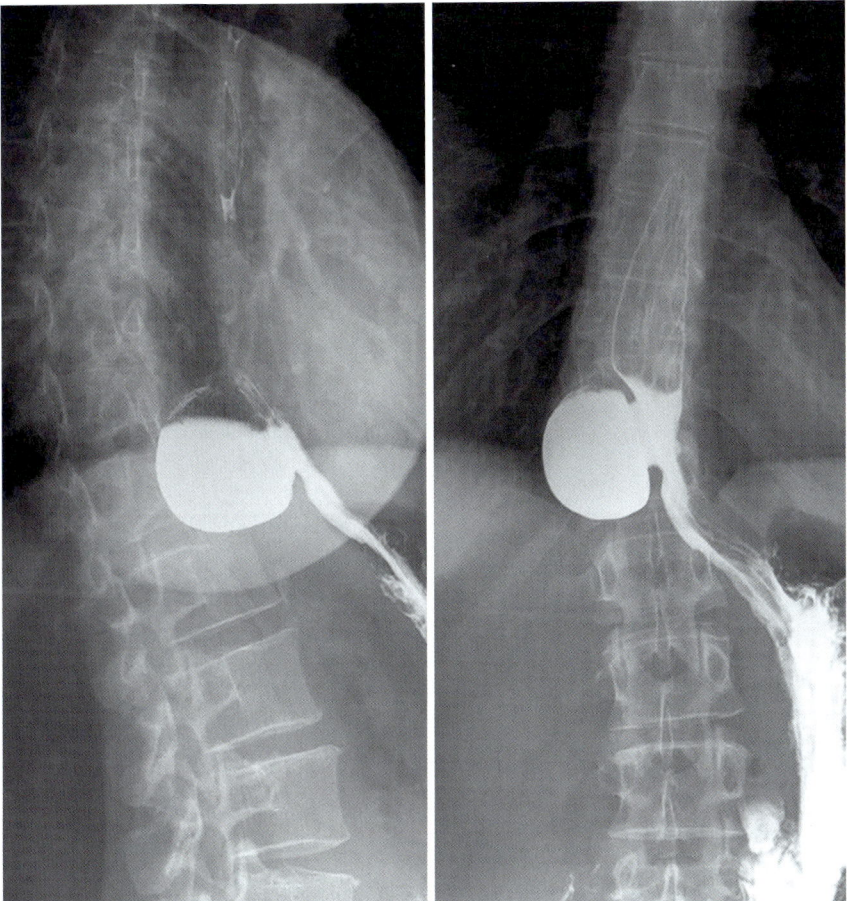

Fig. 20.1 Barium swallow showing a large epiphrenic diverticulum with contrast retention

A timed barium swallow is preferable for the study of the motility disorder. The barium emptying rate, as well as any barium retention with a tortuous esophagus, a "bird-beak" appearance, or an outpouching sac protruding from the esophageal wall, should be recorded (Fig. 20.2).

Upper digestive endoscopy is mandatory in all cases of suspected diverticulum in order to diagnose the diverticulum and rule out malignancy and associated diseases. The examination should be completed after a fast of at least 8 hours (Fig. 20.3). After the food debris or fluid accumulation has been removed, the ED mucosa must be carefully evaluated, and measurements taken of the diverticular neck and its distance from the Z line, in order to properly plan the surgery.

The esophagogastric junction should also be evaluated for any mucosal break suggesting erosive esophagitis, Barrett's esophagus, or hiatal hernia and to evaluate contraction of the lower esophageal sphincter.

Esophageal manometry is performed to identify or confirm the presence of an underlying motility disorder and therefore guide the extension of myotomy during

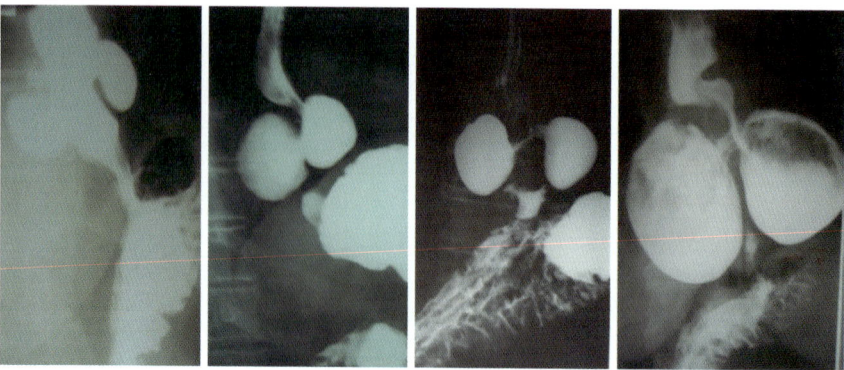

Fig. 20.2 Development over time of a double epiphrenic diverticulum, as shown in sequential barium swallows. Not only is the pouch increasing in size, but there is also evidence of motility dysfunction

Fig. 20.3 Endoscopic view of epiphrenic diverticulum with retention of food debris

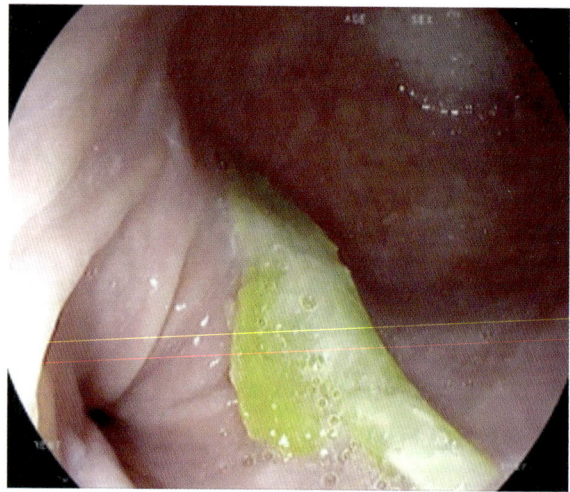

surgery. In cases of symptomatic diverticula, the absence of a clear diagnosis does not exempt from the treatment of the lower esophageal sphincter.

20.5 Indication for Surgery

As the majority of diverticula are discovered incidentally, most of the time endoscopic and clinical observation alone is advisable. When symptoms such as dysphagia and regurgitation are mild or rare, and there are no respiratory complications, surgical treatment is generally not indicated. Careful patient selection is essential as the surgery is complex and can lead to major morbidity mainly due to leakage from the staple line after the diverticulectomy, and the mortality rates are not negligible even in high-volume centers. The size of the diverticulum is not an indication for surgery *per se*, as symptoms are not related to the dimension of diverticula.

20.6 Surgical Approaches

Surgical approaches for ED have evolved from the initial open transthoracic method to the currently preferred abdominal approach, particularly with the advent of laparoscopy. Traditionally, the operation was performed through a left thoracotomy approach and the diverticulectomy was completed with esophago-cardial myotomy and a Belsey Mark IV fundoplication, which is still adopted [11]. Critical aspects of the transthoracic approach regard the postoperative pain and the reduced extension of the myotomy on the gastric side of the cardia. Complication rates following the open transthoracic approach vary from 8.7% to 35.5%, with a leakage rate up to 18.2% [12].

In the early '90 s a minimally invasive approach was proposed, firstly thoracoscopic and then by means of laparoscopy [13–15]. With video-assisted thoracoscopy, myotomy was not performed with an antireflux procedure. Moreover, this procedure still needs single-lung ventilation with placement of a double-lumen orotracheal tube; besides, there was an unfavorable angle between the stapler and the esophageal axis, which caused an imperfect suture line. By contrast, the advantages of a transhiatal laparoscopic approach are to treat the three foundations of ED surgery: treat the diverticular pouch (with perfect placement of the stapler that runs parallel to the esophageal axis), treat the intrinsic motility disorder with a myotomy, and prevent reflux at the same time with a fundoplication. Additionally, laparoscopy allows the myotomy to be extended from the lower esophagus through the stomach and the antireflux surgery to be adapted to the patient's anatomical characteristics. The abdominal approach is also more comfortable for the patients and, as there is no need for transthoracic drains, it is better tolerated in terms of postoperative pain.

In all cases, before surgery it is mandatory for the patient to have a clear liquid diet for at least 24 hours and to fast for at least 12 hours. Depending on the size of the diverticulum, insertion of a double-lumen nasogastric tube 12 hours before surgery to wash and clean the esophageal lumen from food debris is advisable. A rapid sequence intubation is recommended to avoid any inhalation at the time of anesthesia induction.

As in other foregut operations, the patient is placed in the lithotomy position with the surgeon standing between the patient's legs. The cardia and the abdominal esophagus must be completely mobilized, and the esophagus encircled to obtain good traction, taking care not to damage the anterior and posterior vagus nerves. A good exposure of the mediastinal esophagus must be achieved by means of combined blunt and sharp dissection, avoiding pleural tears, which are dangerous for the patient and prevent the surgeon from having adequate vision. This part can be challenging as the diverticulum may be up to 10 cm from the cardia. Intraoperative endoscopy can guide the exposure of the diverticulum, avoiding mucosal injuries

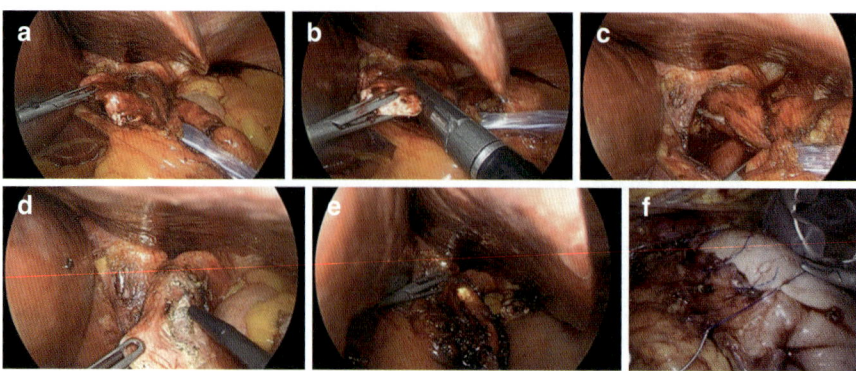

Fig. 20.4 Intraoperative laparoscopic view. (**a**) The diverticulum is dissected from the mediastinum and traction is exerted with neck exposure. (**b**) A linear staple is applied on the diverticular neck, parallel to the esophageal axis. (**c**) The staple line is visible on the lateral part of the esophagus after the diverticulum is transected. (**d**) The second part of surgery comprises the extra-mucosal myotomy. (**e**) After the myotomy has been completed, an endoscopic check is mandatory to assess for any mucosal tear or any bleeding and the residual lumen. (**f**) The last step of surgery involves a fundoplication; in this case an anterior 180° Dor fundoplication has been performed

and helping to safely reach the diverticular neck. Complete dissection of the diverticular neck is mandatory; at its upper angle this might be particularly challenging. After having cleared the diverticular neck, and checked for an adequate lumen of the esophagus, a linear stapler is introduced from a trocar parallel to the esophageal axis and the diverticulum sectioned. A single cartridge is advisable, but not mandatory in the case of long necks.

Then, two or three non-absorbable stitches or a non-absorbable barbed running suture can help close the muscular layer, thus buttressing the mucosal mechanical suture.

The second part of the surgery adds the myotomy of the esophagus, starting from the cardia up to at least the inferior margin of the diverticular neck to aid the bolus transit and avoid overpressure at the level of the staple line, thus reducing staple line leakage. As most diverticula are on the right side of the esophagus, the myotomy should be performed anteriorly or slightly on the left side. After the myotomy is completed, the hiatus is closed with a few braided non-absorbable stitches. Attention must be paid not to narrow the hiatus, resulting in iatrogenic outflow obstruction. The last step of the operation involves the prevention of gastroesophageal reflux, usually with an anterior Dor fundoplication or a posterior Toupet (if a hiatus hernia is present) (Fig. 20.4).

Resolution or decrease in symptoms after laparoscopic surgery are reported in 85–100% [16] of patients, with a leakage rate of 8.8% [7]. Length of stay and postoperative pain is significantly less as compared with the transthoracic approach.

This kind of surgery is not easy and may steps can be tricky, but despite the reported complication and mortality rates, it currently represents the treatment of choice for ED [3, 5, 7]. However, owing to the complexity of the diagnosis and treatment and the possible complications, this surgery should only be performed in high volume centers.

20.7 Endoscopic Treatment

With the growing enthusiasm for endoscopic surgery, more recently peroral endoscopic myotomy with septotomy (D-POEM) has emerged as a therapeutic option. The procedure involves the endoscopic cutting of the muscular fibers of the septum and beyond to the gastroesophageal junction, reached by a submucosal tunnel, to create a common cavity. Very few cases have been reported, but the results have been good in terms of resolution of the symptoms, especially dysphagia [17]. The reported findings of postprocedural radiological examinations, however, seem to show the same anatomical condition, characterized by plenty of contrast medium in the lower esophagus. Furthermore, as for POEM in patients with achalasia, the absence of a fundoplication is associated with a significantly higher reflux. The addition of potential reflux and stasis of food and saliva carries a high risk of damaging the esophageal mucosa.

20.8 Conclusions

Because ED are almost always due an esophageal motility disorder, treatment in most cases must aim to address the motility disorder in addition to resecting the diverticulum. As many of these ED are discovered incidentally, surgery is indicated only for symptomatic patients.

The surgery carries a high rate of complications and the consequences can be fearful with long sequelae and high mortality rates. Different approaches have been illustrated including thoracic, abdominal and even endoscopic approaches but, owing to the small number of reported cases there are no large studies comparing the different techniques.

Laparoscopic transhiatal dissection offers excellent exposure and can be safely performed even in large esophageal diverticula, in tertiary centers with high levels of experience in upper gastrointestinal surgery.

References

1. Thomas ML, Anthony AA, Fosh BG, et al. Oesophageal diverticula. Br J Surg. 2001;88:629–42.
2. Melman L, Quinlan J, Robertson B, et al. Esophageal manometric characteristics and outcomes for laparoscopic esophageal diverticulectomy, myotomy, and partial fundoplication for epiphrenic diverticula. Surg Endosc. 2009;23:1337–41.
3. Rosati R, Fumagalli U, Elmore U, et al. Long-term results of minimally invasive surgery for symptomatic epiphrenic diverticulum. Am J Surg. 2011;201:132–5.

4. Carlson DA, Gluskin AB, Mogni B, et al. Esophageal diverticula are associated with propagating peristalsis: a study utilizing high-resolution manometry. Neurogastroenterol Motil. 2016;28:392–8.
5. Cohen DL, Bermont A, Richter V, et al. Technical success in performing esophageal high-resolution manometry in patients with an epiphrenic diverticulum. Dysphagia. 2024;39:282–8.
6. Triggs JR, Krause AJ, Carlson DA, et al. Blown-out myotomy: an adverse event of laparoscopic Heller myotomy and peroral endoscopic myotomy for achalasia. Gastrointest Endosc. 2021;93:861–868.e1.
7. Herbella FAM, Patti MG. Achalasia and epiphrenic diverticulum. World J Surg. 2015;39:1620–4.
8. Sadasivan CS, Umapathy A. Epiphrenic diverticulum of the oesophagus complicated by the impaction of a foreign body. Thorax. 1962;17:267–70.
9. Dong S, Xie S, Zhou Y. Spontaneous rupture of esophageal diverticulum – a case report and literature review. Diagnostics (Basel). 2022;13:19.
10. Herbella FAM, Dubecz A, Patti MG. Esophageal diverticula and cancer. Dis Esophagus. 2012;25:153–8.
11. Varghese TK Jr, Marshall B, Chang AC, et al. Surgical treatment of epiphrenic diverticula: a 30-year experience. Ann Thorac Surg. 2007;84:1801–9. discussion 1801–9
12. Tapias LF, Morse CR, Mathisen DJ, et al. Surgical management of esophageal epiphrenic diverticula: a transthoracic approach over four decades. Ann Thorac Surg. 2017;104:1123–30.
13. Rosati R, Fumagalli U, Bona S, et al. Laparoscopic treatment of epiphrenic diverticula. J Laparoendosc Adv Surg Tech A. 2001;11:371–5.
14. Rosati R, Fumagalli U, Bona S, et al. Diverticulectomy, myotomy, and fundoplication through laparoscopy: a new option to treat epiphrenic esophageal diverticula? Ann Surg. 1998;227:174–8.
15. Peracchia A, Bonavina L, Rosati R, Bona S. Thoracoscopic resection of epiphrenic diverticula. In: Peters J, DeMeester TR, editors. Minimally invasive surgery of the foregut. St. Louis: QMP Inc.; 1994. p. 110–6.
16. Barbieri LA, Parise P, Cossu A, et al. Treatment of epiphrenic diverticulum: how I do it. J Laparoendosc Adv Surg Tech A. 2020;30:653–8.
17. Nabi Z, Chavan R, Asif S, et al. Per-oral endoscopic myotomy with division of septum (D-POEM) in epiphrenic esophageal diverticula: outcomes at a median follow-up of two years. Dysphagia. 2022;37:839–47.

Open Access This chapter is licensed under the terms of the Creative Commons Attribution-NonCommercial 4.0 International License (http://creativecommons.org/licenses/by-nc/4.0/), which permits any noncommercial use, sharing, adaptation, distribution and reproduction in any medium or format, as long as you give appropriate credit to the original author(s) and the source, provide a link to the Creative Commons license and indicate if changes were made.

The images or other third party material in this chapter are included in the chapter's Creative Commons license, unless indicated otherwise in a credit line to the material. If material is not included in the chapter's Creative Commons license and your intended use is not permitted by statutory regulation or exceeds the permitted use, you will need to obtain permission directly from the copyright holder.

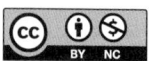

Diffuse Esophageal Spasm

21

Alberto Aiolfi and Davide Bona

21.1 Introduction

Diffuse esophageal spasm (DES) is a motility disorder of the esophagus with no known cause, which can lead to significant discomfort and negatively impact the quality of life for those affected. This condition is marked by irregular smooth muscle contractions in the distal esophagus, resulting in symptoms such as dysphagia, chest pain, and regurgitation. DES is uncommon and challenging to treat, in part due to the limited understanding of its underlying mechanisms. Traditionally, diagnosing DES has depended on subjective symptom assessments and radiographic imaging [1, 2]. However, the introduction of high-resolution manometry (HRM) and the functional lumen imaging probe (FLIP) has allowed for a more precise and objective assessment of esophageal motility disorders, including DES. HRM has become the gold standard for diagnosis, interpreted according to the Chicago Classification (CC). This chapter provides an overview of the current understanding of DES, its clinical presentation, pathophysiology, diagnostic procedures, and management strategies.

21.2 Etiology

The exact cause remains unknown, although several theories have been proposed. One theory suggests that there is a disruption in the coordination of peristalsis, likely due to an imbalance between inhibitory and excitatory postganglionic pathways. Additionally, muscular hypertrophy or hyperplasia can be found in the distal esophagus, affecting nearly two-thirds of it in cases of DES. While the initiating

---

A. Aiolfi (✉) · D. Bona
IRCCS Ospedale Galeazzi – Sant'Ambrogio, Division of General Surgery,
Department of Biomedical Science for Health, University of Milan, Milan, Italy
e-mail: alberto.aiolfi@grupposandonato.it; davide.bona@unimi.it

© The Author(s) 2026
V. Landolfi, S. Tolone (eds.), *Functional Diseases of the Esophagus*, Updates in Surgery, https://doi.org/10.1007/978-3-031-90570-4_21

event is unclear, an increased release of acetylcholine may play a role. Other possible explanations for the peristaltic abnormalities in DES include nitric oxide (NO)-mediated dysfunction of inhibitory ganglion neuronal activity, gastric reflux, or a primary nerve or motor disorder. Furthermore, exposure to acid can lead to esophageal spasms, while heartburn may trigger esophageal contractions. There are also indications that total cholesterol levels and body mass index (BMI) may significantly predict esophageal contractility, and lower esophageal sphincter (LES) function [2–4].

21.3 Epidemiology

The exact prevalence of DES is not well established, as it is a rare condition. Reported prevalence rates vary based on the population studied and the diagnostic criteria applied. Previously known as diffuse esophageal spasm, the condition was reclassified as a distinct diagnosis with the introduction of the CC in 2008. Research suggests that the prevalence of DES among symptomatic patients undergoing esophageal motility testing is approximately 2% to 9%. It tends to occur more frequently in women, with a median age of 60 at the time of diagnosis [3, 4].

21.4 Pathophysiology

DES involves irregular coordination among the smooth muscles of the esophagus, likely resulting from an imbalance between the nitrergic inhibitory and cholinergic excitatory pathways. Typically, there exists a gradual gradient of inhibitory signals from the proximal to distal esophagus, which intensifies as the neuronal signals progress downward. Consequently, the duration of deglutitive inhibition lengthens as the peristaltic wave moves toward the distal esophagus. This period of deglutitive inhibition, known as contractile latency, is considered a defining interval, and a reduction in this interval may lead to premature and rapidly propagating contractions seen in DES. A major focus has been on NO due to its role in the inhibitory pathway of the myenteric plexus. When NO deficiency is induced by scavenger administration, simultaneous esophageal contractions occur, while restoring NO levels can reverse this effect. Opioids, which have been linked to DES, promote NO secretion and inhibit neuronal excitation [1, 2]. In a retrospective study, esophageal dysfunction, such as DES, was found to be more prevalent in individuals using opioids for three months or longer, but these dysfunctions tend to resolve upon discontinuation of the medication [5]. Additionally, almost half of DES patients are reported to take psychotropic medications, suggesting these could also contribute to the disorder. Psychiatric conditions are often associated with chronic pain, potentially leading to excessive opioid use. Gastroesophageal reflux disease (GERD) may also be connected to DES. Abnormal 24-hour pH monitoring is observed in most patients exhibiting GERD symptoms alongside DES, with some reporting symptom relief from antireflux treatments. It is hypothesized that stomach acidity may alter the afferent nerves within the peristaltic peripheral pathways, potentially contributing to DES, though this connection remains debated. Notably, abnormal pH monitoring is primarily associated with typical GERD symptoms rather than chest pain or dysphagia [6]. Spastic achalasia is another condition believed to be pathophysiologically linked to DES. Achalasia is also categorized as a disorder of deglutitive inhibition, with a complete dysfunction of the nitrergic inhibitory pathway in esophageal smooth muscle. Some cases have shown a progression from DES to type 3 achalasia [1].

21.5 Clinical Presentation and Diagnosis

The clinical presentation of DES varies, with symptoms occurring episodically. The most common manifestation is esophageal dysphagia, characterized by difficulty swallowing and/or the sensation of food feeling stuck in the throat or chest. Uncoordinated contractions of the esophagus can also cause retrosternal non-cardiac chest pain, necessitating a preliminary evaluation to rule out acute coronary syndrome. Other associated symptoms include typical and atypical GERD symptoms (such as asthma, coughing, and hoarseness), weight loss, and vomiting. Due to the heterogeneous and non-specific nature of its presentation, diagnosing DES requires specialized testing [7].

Endoscopy is typically the first step to exclude secondary motility disorders (e.g., hiatal hernia, Schatzki's ring, or neoplasms). It also assesses the patency of the LES, aiding in the identification of related conditions, such as achalasia type 3 and GERD. While endoscopy is not used to confirm a DES diagnosis, it may reveal signs of a motility disorder, such as spastic, vigorous, or uncoordinated distal esophageal contractions along with retained saliva or liquid in the esophageal lumen. However, these signs can be easily overlooked due to the sporadic nature of DES [7, 8]. Barium esophagram serves as another complementary diagnostic tool for dysphagia, although its sensitivity for detecting motility disorders is less than 70%. A classic finding in this test is the "corkscrew" or "rosary bead" appearance [8].

The gold standard for diagnosis is HRM, interpreted using the standardized CC system. In the latest version (v 4.0), DES is defined as the presence of premature contractions in at least 20% of swallows, occurring alongside normal LES relaxation in individuals experiencing dysphagia or non-cardiac chest pain. This distinction is noteworthy compared to the previous CC version, which did not require relevant esophageal symptoms. CC v4.0 also acknowledges that intrabolus pressure on HRM can lead to the overdiagnosis of DES. This pressure can be distinguished from true contractile activity by its more homogeneous appearance on Clouse plots and through adjustments to the isobaric contour [9–14]. Premature contractions are characterized by a distal latency (DL) of less than 4.5 seconds. DL is measured from the onset of upper esophageal sphincter relaxation to the contractile deceleration point (CDP) of the peristaltic wave, which is normally located 2–3 cm above the LES. The CDP indicates the transition from esophageal peristaltic clearance to esophageal emptying, identifiable where the pressure curve slope shifts from positive to negative. Normal LES relaxation is defined by an integrated relaxation pressure (IRP) of 15 mmHg or less. It is important to note that DL can be inaccurately low in cases of large hernias due to overall shortening of the esophagus. In order to increase both sensitivity and specificity in inconclusive cases, provocative maneuvers in the supine (multiple rapid swallows [MRS]) and upright (rapid drink challenge [RDC]) have been included in CC v4.0. The goal of MRS is to evaluate the peristaltic reserve of the esophagus by stimulating a rapid series of repetitive contractions, based on the hypothesis of progressively falling esophageal inhibition. RDC can detect esophagogastric junction (EGJ) obstruction and esophageal shortening that can be found in achalasia and other motility disorders [7, 8].

While HRM remains the gold standard, a newer modality called FLIP is being increasingly utilized as a complementary tool in evaluating esophageal motility. FLIP assesses esophageal luminal diameter and distensibility using impedance planimetry. Its catheter includes a distal pressure calculator and multiple impedance sensors surrounded by a distensible balloon. The catheter is inserted either nasally or orally down to the EGJ where it is inflated, generating a radial force against the esophageal wall. Data is analyzed in real time and displayed as distensibility index (DI) and EGJ diameter. DI is the ratio of the EGJ cross-sectional area to intraballoon pressure and is normally >2.0 mm^2/mmHg, while the EGJ diameter is >13 mm. DI is often low in DES, indicating low compliance of the esophagus, while EGJ diameter tends to be normal or slightly reduced [11–13]. FLIP can also topographically display secondary peristalsis from balloon distension as anterograde or retrograde contractions in the esophageal body. Repetitive retrograde contractions or sustained occluding contractions secondary to balloon distension can be encountered in DES [10]. FLIP might better detect secondary peristalsis when compared to HRM, as its catheter is less contact-dependent and can detect non-lumen-occluding contractions [13]. The data by FLIP can be objectively interpreted in real time, is less operator dependent, and allows for a more complete picture of esophageal physiology as compared to HRM. It can also predict the clinical outcomes of myotomy, whether done surgically or endoscopically [14]. The data on the LES makes FLIP particularly useful in the evaluation of achalasia and esophagogastric junction outflow obstruction (EGJ-OO), as these may be associated with DES [1].

21.6 Treatment

Due to the unclear pathophysiology of DES, treatment can be challenging. Both pharmacologic and invasive approaches have been developed, primarily aimed at relieving symptoms rather than normalizing manometric findings.

21.6.1 Proton-Pump Inhibitors (PPIs)

Many patients with DES experience reflux-like symptoms, and GERD may coexist with DES. Abnormal 24-hour pH monitoring is often observed in patients with

21 Diffuse Esophageal Spasm

esophageal hypomotility. Therefore, a trial of PPIs is recommended if GERD is likely, while pH testing off PPIs may be warranted if GERD is unlikely [7].

21.6.2 Smooth Muscle Relaxants

Smooth muscle relaxants can help alleviate symptoms. Nitrates and phosphodiesterase-5 inhibitors (PDE5i) work by increasing NO availability, promoting smooth muscle relaxation. Long-acting nitrates, such as isosorbide dinitrate, are effective for non-cardiac chest pain and dysphagia when taken about 30 minutes before meals. Calcium-channel blockers (CCBs) also induce relaxation by inhibiting L-type calcium channels. Sublingual nifedipine is effective but has a shorter duration compared to nitrates. In a clinical trial, sildenafil (50 mg) showed manometric improvement in most patients, although symptomatic relief was limited [15].

21.6.3 Peppermint Oil

Peppermint oil has been shown to relax gastrointestinal smooth muscle by reducing extracellular calcium influx. Studies indicate that it can eliminate simultaneous esophageal contractions in DES patients. In one study, most patients with DES reported symptomatic improvement after using peppermint oil [16].

Overall, pharmacologic therapies have limited utility due to their variable efficacy, the need for frequent dosing, side effects, and inadequate clinical trial support. If pharmacologic management fails, more invasive options may be considered.

21.6.4 Botulinum Toxin Injection

Botulinum toxin is a powerful neurotoxin that induces reversible chemical denervation and partial paralysis by inhibiting the presynaptic release of acetylcholine in muscle fibers. It has been established as an effective short-term treatment for achalasia, particularly in medically high-risk patients. However, the evidence for using botulinum toxin injections to treat non-achalasia esophageal motility disorders, such as DES, is inconsistent. When used for these disorders, the primary target symptom is likely dysphagia, and there is data supporting the use of injections into both the distal esophagus and the LES [17].

21.6.5 Peroral Endoscopic Myotomy (POEM)

POEM is a novel intervention primarily designed for treating achalasia and other esophageal motility disorders. While it has predominantly been studied in the context of achalasia, recent investigations have explored its use for non-achalasia spastic esophageal motility disorders, including DES. A meta-analysis of five studies focusing on outcomes of POEM in non-achalasia esophageal disorders, including DES, showed promising clinical success lasting beyond 60 months. However, some case reports and series on POEM's efficacy for non-achalasia conditions have either unclear follow-up periods or short-term data, raising concerns about publication bias. Given the generally benign nature of primary esophageal motility disorders like DES and the lack of robust studies on the safety and efficacy of invasive methods like POEM, the European Society of Gastrointestinal Endoscopy recommends caution regarding its use [1, 18, 19]. POEM should be considered when medical and less invasive treatments fail, especially in patients experiencing severe dysphagia that leads to weight loss.

21.6.6 Surgery

Surgery is generally reserved for cases of refractory and severe DES, as the prognosis for DES is typically favorable even without intervention [8, 20, 21]. Extended myotomy combined with anterior fundoplication for DES have been shown to result in significant chest pain and dysphagia score improvements in the long-term follow-up.

21.7 Take Home Message

DES is a rare motility disorder characterized by premature contractions of the distal esophageal smooth muscle. The pathophysiology likely involves an imbalance between the inhibitory and excitatory pathways of the smooth muscles. Diagnosing DES is challenging due to its variable and episodic symptoms. HRM is currently the gold standard for diagnosis and is interpreted using the CC. Recent updates to the CC have improved the accuracy of the diagnosis, including the incorporation of provocative maneuvers and the differentiation of DES from achalasia type 3. FLIP is a newer modality that provides complementary information to HRM, allowing for a more comprehensive evaluation of esophageal motility. Managing DES is difficult due to the limited understanding of its pathophysiology. Treatment options include PPIs for concurrent GERD symptoms, smooth muscle relaxants such as nitrates and CCBs, and peppermint oil. However, pharmacological therapy has limited efficacy and frequent dosing requirements. Endoscopic approaches such as botulinum toxin injection and POEM or surgical myotomy may be considered in patients with recalcitrant symptoms.

References

1. Gorti H, Samo S, Shahnavaz N, Qayed E. Distal esophageal spasm: update on diagnosis and management in the era of high-resolution manometry. World J Clin Cases. 2020;8(6):1026–32.
2. Khalaf M, Chowdhary S, Elias PS, Castell D. Distal esophageal spasm: a review. Am J Med. 2018;131(9):1034–40.

3. Pandolfino JE, Roman S, Carlson D, et al. Distal esophageal spasm in high-resolution esophageal pressure topography: defining clinical phenotypes. Gastroenterology. 2011;141(2):469–75.
4. Almansa C, Heckman MG, DeVault KR, et al. Esophageal spasm: demographic, clinical, radiographic, and manometric features in 108 patients. Dis Esophagus. 2012;25(3):214–21.
5. Snyder DL, Crowell MD, Horsley-Silva J, et al. Opioid-induced esophageal dysfunction: differential effects of type and dose. Am J Gastroenterol. 2019;114(9):1464–9.
6. Crespin OM, Tatum RP, Yates RB, et al. Esophageal hypermotility: cause or effect? Dis Esophagus. 2016;29(5):497–502.
7. Roman S, Hebbard G, Jung KW, et al. Chicago Classification Update (v4.0): technical review on diagnostic criteria for distal esophageal spasm. Neurogastroenterol Motil. 2021;33(5):e14119.
8. Patel DA, Yadlapati R, Vaezi MF. Esophageal motility disorders: current approach to diagnostics and therapeutics. Gastroenterology. 2022;162(6):1617–34.
9. Sharma P, Yadlapati R. Evaluation of esophageal motility and lessons from Chicago Classification version 4.0. Curr Gastroenterol Rep. 2022;24(1):10–7.
10. Sirinawasatien A, Sakulthongthawin P. Manometrically jackhammer esophagus with fluoroscopically/endoscopically distal esophageal spasm: a case report. BMC Gastroenterol. 2021;21(1):222.
11. Bredenoord AJ, Rancati F, Lin H, et al. Normative values for esophageal functional lumen imaging probe measurements: a meta-analysis. Neurogastroenterol Motil. 2022;34(11):e14419.
12. Carlson DA, Baumann AJ, Prescott JE, et al. Validation of secondary peristalsis classification using FLIP panometry in 741 subjects undergoing manometry. Neurogastroenterol Motil. 2022;34(1):e14192.
13. Chen HM, Li BW, Li LY, et al. Functional lumen imaging probe in gastrointestinal motility diseases. J Dig Dis. 2019;20(11):572–7.
14. Yadlapati R, Kahrilas PJ, Fox MR, et al. Esophageal motility disorders on high-resolution manometry: Chicago classification version 4.0©. Neurogastroenterol Motil. 2021;33(1):e14058.
15. Bortolotti M, Mari C, Lopilato C, et al. Effects of sildenafil on esophageal motility of patients with idiopathic achalasia. Gastroenterology. 2000;118(2):253–7.
16. Pimentel M, Bonorris GG, Chow EJ, Lin HC. Peppermint oil improves the manometric findings in diffuse esophageal spasm. J Clin Gastroenterol. 2001;33(1):27–31.
17. Bashashati M, Andrews C, Ghosh S, Storr M. Botulinum toxin in the treatment of diffuse esophageal spasm. Dis Esophagus. 2010;23(7):554–60.
18. Weusten BLAM, Barret M, Bredenoord AJ, et al. Endoscopic management of gastrointestinal motility disorders – Part 1: European Society of Gastrointestinal Endoscopy (ESGE) Guideline. Endoscopy. 2020;52(6):498–515.
19. Nabi Z, Mandavdhare H, Akbar W, et al. Long-term outcome of peroral endoscopic myotomy in esophageal motility disorders: a systematic review and meta-analysis. J Clin Gastroenterol. 2023;57(3):227–38.
20. Aiolfi A, Bona D, Riva CG, et al. Systematic review and bayesian network meta-analysis comparing laparoscopic Heller myotomy, pneumatic dilatation, and peroral endoscopic myotomy for esophageal achalasia. J Laparoendosc Adv Surg Tech A. 2020;30(2):147–55.
21. Almansa C, Hinder RA, Smith CD, Achem SR. A comprehensive appraisal of the surgical treatment of diffuse esophageal spasm. J Gastrointest Surg. 2008;12:1133–45.

Open Access This chapter is licensed under the terms of the Creative Commons Attribution-NonCommercial 4.0 International License (http://creativecommons.org/licenses/by-nc/4.0/), which permits any noncommercial use, sharing, adaptation, distribution and reproduction in any medium or format, as long as you give appropriate credit to the original author(s) and the source, provide a link to the Creative Commons license and indicate if changes were made.

The images or other third party material in this chapter are included in the chapter's Creative Commons license, unless indicated otherwise in a credit line to the material. If material is not included in the chapter's Creative Commons license and your intended use is not permitted by statutory regulation or exceeds the permitted use, you will need to obtain permission directly from the copyright holder.

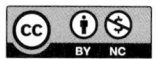